THE

An Average Joe's Path to Balancing Family, Work, and Triathlon

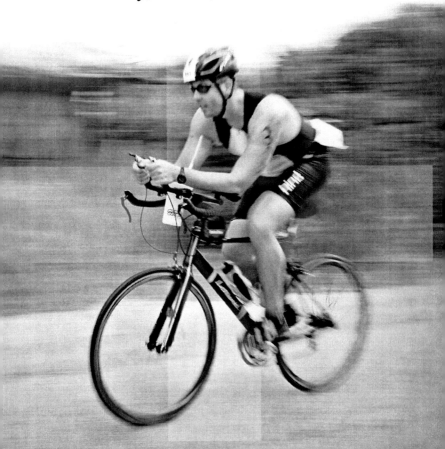

DAVID MILLS

2.4 MILE SWIM | 112 MILE BIKE | 26.2 MILE RUN

THE DISTANCE

An Average Joe's Path to Balancing Family, Work and Triathlon
by David G. Mills

ISBN: 978-1-935986-10-2

TheAverageIronman@gmail.com

www.TheDistanceBook.com

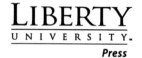

Press

Lynchburg, VA

www.liberty.edu/libertyuniversitypress

{ DEDICATION }

This book is dedicated to my sons, Luke and Braeden. The world will be a better place because of men like you leading in the next generation. Dream BIG. Go BIG. I can't wait to see what great things God has planned for your lives. You were my inspiration throughout all of my training and racing. You're the kind of sons that every guy in this world hopes to have. I thank God that I'm the one blessed with the task of being your dad.

And to my parents, for always getting me the right gear and shoes (and knee surgeries) for every sport I ever played growing up, for traveling to all of my games, and for ceaselessly praying for me throughout my entire life. Rain or shine, I've always known that I'd see you standing there, waiting for me at the finish line.

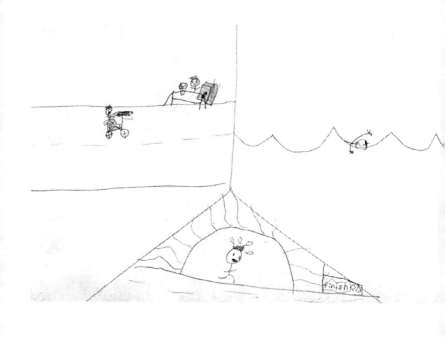

{ I PROMISED MY SON IF I EVER WROTE A BOOK THAT I'D LET HIM ILLUSTRATE IT. SO HERE IS LUKE'S TRIATHLON ART WORK. }

{ EXPLANATION }

An Ironman, while it is the most well known, is just one of many full-distance triathlons around the world. The term full-distance refers to any triathlon that is 140.6 miles in duration – with a 2.4-mile swim, 112-mile bike and 26.2-mile run. These are sometimes called ultra-distance or iron-distance races. The Revolution 3 Triathlon Race Series, which focuses on a fun spectator experience for the whole family, refers to them as "full Rev." The website www.irondistance.com provides a comprehensive list of incredible full-distance triathlons around the world. Beach to Battleship in Wilmington, N.C., and Nevada's Silverman are just two examples of great full-distance triathlons. The term Ironman is simply the registered trademark of the World Triathlon Corporation, and while the event described in this book is the Louisville Ironman, the information and inspiration is certainly not limited to just a single trademark. This book is for all full-distance triathletes (especially those who aren't sure if they can do it).

{ CONTENTS }

Preface   The Average Joe 9

Introduction   By Jeffrey Jeffords..................................... 11

Chapter 1   The Big Question...................................... 17

Chapter 2   The Background 23

Chapter 3   The Compromise 29

Chapter 4   The Moon 37

Chapter 5   The Excuse 41

Chapter 6   The Calling 47

Chapter 7   The Everyman 55

Chapter 8   The Family 61

Chapter 9   The Job 75

Chapter 10   The Swim 83

Chapter 11   The Bike 95

Chapter 12   The Run 113

Chapter 13   The Setback 123

Chapter 14   The Aid Station 131

Chapter 15   The Taper 137

Chapter 16   The Transition 145

Chapter 17   The Travel 151

Chapter 18   The Race 159

Chapter 19   The Aftermath 181

Acknowledgements 185

About The Author 187

{ PREFACE }
THE AVERAGE JOE

"God must love the common man. He made so many of them." —
Abraham Lincoln

So, you're thinking about doing an Ironman. Or maybe you're just trying to understand why on earth your friend or spouse wants to attempt one. You're flipping through this book and it's on a shelf with a lot of other books, books that are written by professional athletes, trainers, coaches, or people with Ph.D.s in Exercise Physiology. That's all well and good if you have a personal chef, a masseuse and 30 hours a week to train. Those books have a lot of great things in them. They will explain to you the process of your body building mitochondria as you train. Those books will explain the subtle differences between VO2 max and anaerobic threshold. I've read those books and they really are good — you might even find something in them that's useful.

But the book that you're holding right now has something that those other books don't — a life. This book was written by a guy who worked crazy long hours flying jets in the Air Force, went on weekly dates with his wife to keep the romance alive, played and read with his kids everyday, took night classes for a master's degree and still managed to train for an Ironman! This book is written by a regular-looking guy.

A guy who could stand to lose 10 pounds. A guy who had to change poopy diapers before his bike rides. A guy who made pancakes for his kids in the morning before he went running. A guy who was afraid of a speedo! And this guy can tell you how it can be done.

So you've got a bad knee and a gut, maybe you work long hours on swing shifts or maybe you're terrible at swimming. Well, I do too. But I can explain how I balanced it all – God, family, work, training and how to become a better person as a result. You will walk away from this book feeling motivated and encouraged. You will be informed about just how much training is enough to cross that finish line, and you'll benefit from lots of practical tips.

This is my candid story of an Average Joe who simply decided to go all out. If you've ever wondered if you could do an Ironman then this book is for you. You won't have to quit your job or forsake your family. In fact, training for and finishing an Ironman might just make you better in other areas of your life.

If you only read one book in preparation for your Ironman make it the one by the guy who knows you've got more going on in your life than just training. I understand the sacrifice, the time, travel, money and emotions involved in chasing down the Ironman dream. Let this book prepare and equip you for the 140.6-mile event that will change your life.

(Understanding lactic acid buildup is fun, but it won't really help you any.)

{ INTRODUCTION }
BY JEFFERY JEFFORDS

Every now and again, someone shares a chapter of his or her life with us over a cup of coffee and it just resonates. That's what happened when my friend David began sharing his journey with me, a journey that he made from Average Joe to Ironman. David's story of commitment and perseverance is relevant to anyone who wants to do significant things, but not at the expense of the most important things in life. David's story is a must read for the Ironman-in-training, and a compelling read for anyone who wants to unleash their inner-Ironman in pursuit of significant dreams. Make no mistake — David was inspired by a dream rather than a common goal. David's pursuit was of the creative, soul-stirring, entrepreneurial, passionate realm. I was moved by this story and I was reminded that real people can do amazing things when they work hard, think strategically and exercise faith.

David's story to go The Distance is engaging, entertaining and challenging, while also offering practical insights for those with Ironman aspirations. What engrossed me in his story, however, was the richness of the life applications. As I read about David pushing through barriers and remaining focused on his big dream, I found myself processing the relevant parallels to my own work life, family life and spiritual life. David didn't simply endeavor to complete a task at any cost, he had the courage to follow his dream in the right way and in the right time. That's a pursuit that we all should share; we should pursue worthy endeavors, push through obstacles and chase our dreams with integrity and passion.

As a church planter, I was able to relate David's journey to a different context of life. As David trained for his Ironman competition while in Okinawa, Japan, I was halfway around the world preparing to launch a new church. When David began to share the nature of his Ironman journey with me, I was astounded by the similarity of the obstacles that we each had faced on our completely different, yet remarkably similar journeys. My church-planting journey was stretching me and growing my faith as David's Ironman journey was having the same effect on his life. Even more coincidentally, we learned that David and I shared an affinity for the same leadership podcasts and messages from Pastor Andy Stanley that we often listened to during our training. To be sure, it was a providential connection.

Anytime a person decides to dream big and go after a big goal, it will inspire the people around him. That's how David's desire to become an Ironman was born. It was a friend that inspired him and exposed him to the "Ironman bug." It's amazing how a friend can challenge us to stretch ourselves. I love that the defining nature of the friends we choose is so embedded in David's story and that it culminates in such a profound way. As David's journey towards becoming an Ironman unfolds, we can sense the relational influence of his friend Lance and the camaraderie of the Ironman community. Friends listen to your dreams, they have faith in you and they encourage you to face down obstacles. Encouragement becomes something more than casual conversation when a courageous friend realizes his own dream and challenges us to do the same. When an accomplished friend believes in us, it fuels our soul and empowers our dreams.

At the center of David's life, we find that he's a Godly guy who earnestly seeks to put first things first. David has a fantastic family and a successful career in the Air Force as a navigator, but we discover that like us, David struggles to balance family, career and the rest of life's pursuits. David recognized that training for an Ironman would impact his family life. David knew that at least in some small ways, his family would have to make sacrifices to support him. The creative and intentional ways that David involves his family in his training, along with the love and support shown by his wife Kerry, is inspiring. He shows us that it's possible to remain fully engaged with one's family and do your job well while training for an Ironman. Balancing your life isn't easy, but we can learn some things from David's story as he learned to prioritize well and lean in to family in the right moments.

The training regimen that David develops certainly draws upon the experience of others, but he adds his own practical solutions. David was always thinking about steps and solutions to tackle the rigors of training for an Ironman. David trained physically, mentally and spiritually. David considered how he would feel mentally when race day came, and he prepared for it in creative ways. His vision for utilizing the aid stations in the race reflects how our Heavenly Father restores and refuels us. David set short-term goals that strategically supported his long-term goal. David found the time to train using outside-the-box thinking and he accomplished something that many of us repeatedly fail at. He refused to quit on a worthwhile dream when things got tough.

David's Ironman race itself offers such a compelling conclusion to this story. Anything worth doing is going to call upon the fortitude to push through obstacles. In many cases, obstacles are quite tangible things, but at the end of the day, they all become mental. Training for an Ironman is quite the physical challenge. David says that 90 percent of this epic task is the training and 10 percent is the event itself, but 100 percent of the emotion is unleashed on race day. When you read this book, you're going to feel the emotion and you'll find yourself pulling for my friend David to fulfill his Ironman dream. You'll swim alongside him, you'll ride with him on his bike and you'll run in his shoes as you take part in a grueling race and march towards the finish line. You'll dream big again.

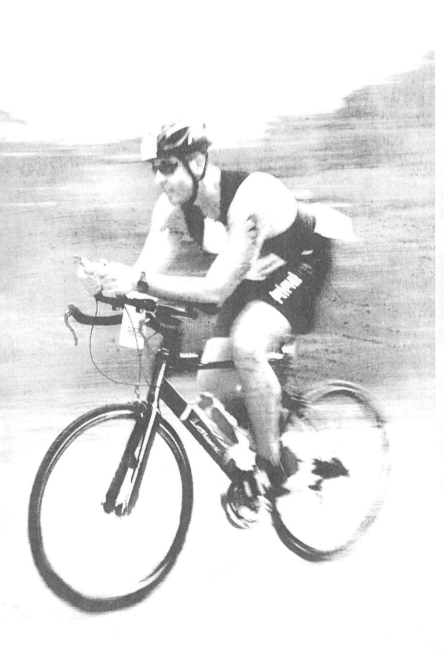

CHAPTER 1

THE BIG QUESTION

"In any moment of decision, the best thing you can do is the right thing, the next best thing is the wrong thing, and the worst thing you can do is nothing." — Theodore Roosevelt

There is something deep inside all of us that asks the question, "Could I do that?" We see other human beings doing it. We cannot help but wonder if they possess something that we do not. Are they special? Are they unique? What about me? Am I not made of the same material? Could I do this thing? Could I become an Ironman? Let me caution you right there — if you are asking yourself that question then, my friend, you have already been infected with the Ironman bug. And once that happens there is only one way to cure it. You have to answer the question. You have to know. You have to find out if you can do it. You have to test yourself.

I can't believe how many times I've heard people say, "I could never do that." I want to say, "Of course not; you haven't trained for it yet." That's like thinking, "I could never land an airplane." Well you could if you were trained for it, and went through flight school. Or, "I could never play the piano." Well, you could if you practiced. The Ironman is no different. No one is expected to be able to swim well the very first time they jump in one of the lanes at their local YMCA pool, or ride 100 miles when they get on a bike for the first time since they were a kid.

It takes training. It takes patience. But absolutely anyone can do it if they have a strong enough desire.

An Ironman is not made on race day. It is not the day of the event that requires the enormous amount of endurance and perseverance. It is the 13 grueling months prior to the day of the race that require these attributes. Race day is simply the culmination. Race day is your celebration and public display of the training you've already done. An Ironman is not made on race day amongst the crowds and cheers and volunteers. An Ironman is made on the lonely streets of your own town, and the cold swimming pool just down the street. An Ironman is made in training.

"Could I do that?"

That was the phrase that I could not get out of my head as I stood in Madison, Wisconsin in 2006. It was raining as I stood there watching the finishers cross the finish line. It was my first-ever experience with an Ironman and I was cheering on two of my friends from Omaha, Nebraska. They were, in my opinion, crazy. In fact, I couldn't imagine that I actually even *knew* someone attempting an Ironman. It had never even so much as crossed my mind that one day I might be the one in the race. I stood on the water's edge completely in awe as I heard the cannon fire and watched over 2,000 people start the swim at 7 a.m. The energy in the air was almost tangible. The atmosphere was electric. There was more human emotion in the air than I'd ever witnessed before at any sporting event. The rest of the day only got more intense.

If you've never before watched an Ironman in person, you are missing out on the most exciting sport in existence. (This is a proven scientific fact and in no way an exaggeration). As the night gets later and the midnight cutoff approaches, the tension peaks. Standing at the finish line in Madison, I watched as hundreds of folks poured across the finish line in a steady stream that went on for hours. Some of them did cartwheels. Some cheered. Some cried. There were those who limped, those who sprinted and those who puked. Some looked elated and others looked half-dead. I could not look away. These people had been swimming, biking and running for nearly 17 hours. The professionals that won had long since showered, eaten dinner, and gone to bed. But for the Average Joes still out there on the course, the day was still far from over. I watched dumbfounded as fit 20-something's failed to finish in time, as senior citizens completed the race, and as wives, husbands and children hugged and cheered with their family members as the announcer proclaimed, "You are an Ironman!" It was fantastic. It was the greatest show on earth and it didn't even charge the spectators for admission.

It set the bar high for sporting events, and ever since I've been unable to care about the World Series or the Super Bowl, all of which are now mere smoke and lights with silly half time shows and seventh inning stretches. No one blacks out, pukes, or crawls to the finish line. All I see is million-dollar deals, commercial breaks and timeouts. These are not sports. These are just games. I had been spoiled by what I'd seen; I had become infected with the Ironman bug. As I watched the show of human emotion spill itself over the finish line, I heard the phrase in the back of my mind, and I asked that question for the first time.

"Could I do that?"

At first I dismissed the question entirely. There were plenty of distractions in my life, such as family and work, that I could use to help silence that haunting question. These were noble distractions. Certainly no one would think less of me for focusing on family and work instead of chasing an endurance event that is certifiably beyond all reason or good sense.

For billions of fortunate people in the world, that seems to be sufficient. They are able to move on and live their lives and forget about the question, or maybe they are blissfully unaware that the question even exists. "Could I do that?" Unfortunately, I was not in that blissful majority that remains immune to the Ironman fever and its haunting, infectious question. "Could I do that?" I was, unfortunately, in the very small minority that must (for better or worse) have that question answered.

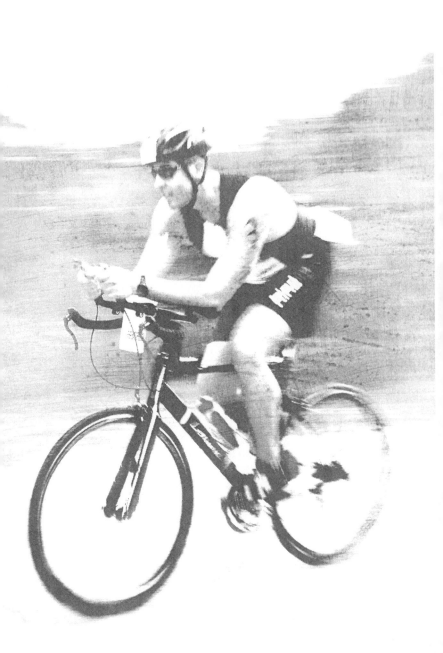

CHAPTER 2

THE BACKGROUND

"Some people consider the marathon the ultimate endurance event.
We consider it a cool down." — Unknown

You know that any sport that was invented by a group of Navy SEALs over a bet is going to be one tough sport. Even its name is cool — Ironman. If you can even finish the thing you earn the title Ironman and enter a small fraternity of Ironman finishers.

As the story goes, US Navy Officer, John Collins, founded the Ironman in Hawaii in 1977, over a friendly debate about who was the most fit, the swimmer, cyclist, or runner. The wager was thrown out that whoever could complete the Waikiki Rough Water Swim (2.4 miles), the Around-Oahu Bike Race (originally a two-day event) and the Honolulu Marathon — all three without a break in between — would be the most fit.

The group agreed, and on February 18, 1978, 15 men participated in the first-ever Ironman Triathlon. Only 12 of those men would finish the race. The winner was Gordon Haller (US Navy) with a time of 11 hours, 46 minutes. The runner up, a US Navy SEAL named John Dunbar, had famously run out of water during the run and had been drinking only beer!

The race continued each year, and each year more and more people showed up for it. Word of the race spread, it wasn't heavily advertised and it wasn't broadcasted. It was whispered about, and rumored. It was an underground event for the borderline insane and the truly masochistic.

Soon enough, Sports Illustrated, wrote a piece about the event and its popularity began to grow. Then in 1982, CBS caught the remarkable finish of Julie Moss on their Wide World of Sports, and the infamy of the sport swept across the globe. Moss collapsed from fatigue and dehydration just a few yards away from crossing the finish line. Television viewers everywhere held their breath as Moss stumbled to get back up. She was just yards away from being the first-place female. As she stumbled and fell yet again she was passed by Kathleen McCartney, but for some reason it was Moss that the cameras followed. A semi-coherent Moss resigned to her knees, her legs no longer willing to cooperate, began to crawl to the finish line. In one of the most gut-wrenching finishes in the world of sports, Julie Moss crawled across the finish line on her hands and knees. In that moment, the world witnessed the sheer guts and tenacity possessed by the Ironman.

{ **TIP: DON'T GET A $500 AERO HELMET IF YOU KNOW IT'S GOING TO TAKE YOU SEVEN HOURS TO FINISH THE BIKE.** }

From 15 participants in 1978 to 44,000 in 2009, the Ironman Triathlon has spread like wildfire. There are events held all around the world from Singapore, Japan and Australia, to Arizona and Kentucky.

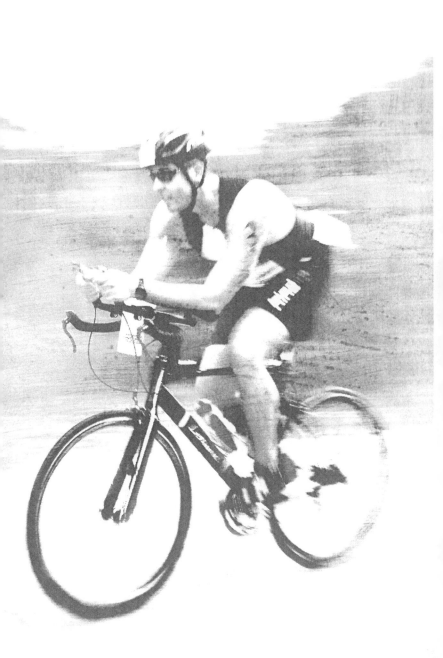

CHAPTER 3

THE COMPROMISE

"Twenty years from now you will be more disappointed by the things that you didn't do than by the ones you did do." — Mark Twain

One year after witnessing the Madison Ironman I thought that I had cured myself of Ironman fever. I had managed to dismiss the question and move on with life. Still, I thought often about the way U2's song, Beautiful Day, blasted over the speakers at the race start and how I felt impotent standing there on the shore holding my cup of coffee. Smug. Comfortable. About 2,000 folks more daring and adventurous than myself (not too mention much older — I was a spry 27-year-old at the time) plunged into the cold water. Less than 17 hours later, each finisher was dubbed an Ironman. I was dubbed a spectator.

Like so many millions of others, I found the perfect way to cure myself of the Ironman bug without actually having to do an Ironman. I found the perfect compromise. A marathon. That was it! It was the perfect answer. Running a marathon was acceptable. It was sane. It was popular. It was trendy. It was hip. Everybody runs a marathon these days. The distinguished list of marathon runners includes everyone from Will Ferrell and Dana Carvey to George W. Bush and Al Gore. David Lee Roth and Sean "P Diddy" Combs have run marathons. Oprah ran one for crying out loud. Is there anyone who has not run a marathon?

So I decided to register for a marathon. This would be a real endurance race, right? This would help me answer that question that had pestered me since Madison.

Training for a marathon is challenging, but training for one during a Nebraska winter is just no fun at all. I remember training for the 2007 Lincoln Nebraska marathon in the piercing cold wind on Omaha's Keystone Trail. This flat and desolate trail has nothing around to break the wind. There's no trees, buildings or hills. The trail runs through flat fields and completely exposes those who travel it to the driving winds of the plains. I was wearing the pants from a warm up suit, a hooded sweatshirt, wool cap and gloves. My buddy was dressed in similar attire, plus he was wearing ski goggles. This was actually a pretty good idea. Although it looked ridiculous and brought a few good laughs, it did manage to keep his eyeballs from drying out and freezing in the open position. This was a problem I learned all about. Soon enough, I would be unable to see how silly he looked.

After about five or six miles into our run, I realized that I had much bigger problems than my eyes. There was a freezing pain between my legs that was becoming increasingly difficult to ignore. Beneath my jogging pants were only my cotton boxers. These offered zero protection from the assault of wind and blowing snow. I took off one of my gloves, stuffed it down my pants and used it as an extra layer down there. So now he's running with ski goggles and I'm wearing only one glove. Things soon got worse. If I were foolish for not wearing warmer underwear, then my buddy was equally as guilty of another rookie mistake.

Now if you've never run more than 10 or 12 miles before you might not be aware of the important role that band aids play when it comes to your nipples. But on that day as we jogged along for 15 miles and my buddy's shirt rubbed and chaffed against his very cold chest, he learned this lesson the hard way (so to speak). And reminiscent of my outburst at mile five, my buddy starts frantically removing his fleece, then his T-shirt, then his thermal shirt. Now it's about 10 degrees

{ **TIP: DON'T TIE YOUR SHOES TOO TIGHT. YOUR FEET WILL SWELL A LOT DURING A 15+ MILE RUN.** }

outside and he's running proudly bare chested, dried blood coming down from his nipples, and wearing ski goggles. About every mile or so, I take my one glove off and put in on the other hand. I'm sure we looked like a pair of real pro athletes in training.

It was hard and it was a challenging. There's nothing easy about choosing to ruin a perfectly good Saturday with an 18-mile training run. It was hard. Do not get me wrong. Training for a marathon is not something to be taken lightly, and anyone who finishes one has certainly displayed some dedication, endurance, discipline and willpower.

For some reason, however, I felt strangely unfulfilled upon completing a marathon. The sense of pride that I had anticipated wasn't there. I felt a let down. It was anticlimactic. The other runners were in their own worlds just as I was. I listened to my iPod the entire time just like most of the others. I had built an impressive playlist and I rocked out the entire time. There were way less fans than I had expected. I remember passing the half-way marker and the runners who were only doing the half-marathon were walking toward their cars with their medals around their necks. All were strangely quiet. They just headed to their cars, maybe to go run some errands. They seemed oblivious to the guy jogging by them that still had another 13 miles to go. We had nothing in common that day other than our free T-shirts. There was no real bond or sense of community that comes about when you and a complete stranger both suffer together.

My mind went back to that previous year in Madison, Wisconsin, where I had witnessed that shared experience that united all those strangers together. They had cheered each other on, even as they were passing another racer. There was something about that Ironman that I could not really define or quite put my finger on. But I had witnessed its energy, and it made me aware that something was noticeably missing from this marathon. I plodded on for the second half and I finished. Then I drove home to run some errands.

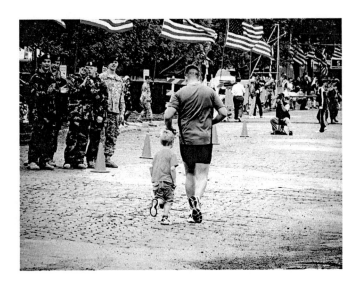

Crossing the finish line of the Lincoln Nebraska Marathon in 2007 with my son Luke.

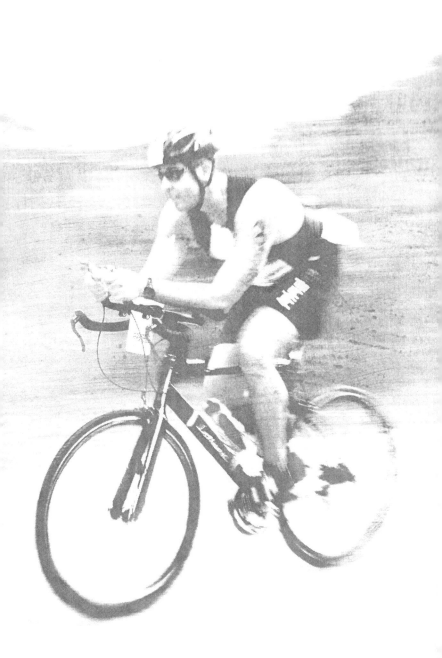

CHAPTER 4

THE MOON

It's faith in something and enthusiasm for something that makes a life worth living. — Oliver Wendell Holmes

There is a great old Saturday Night Live sketch that portrays an older Neil Armstrong walking through a supermarket doing his grocery shopping. In the sketch you can hear Armstrong's inner thoughts, and all that the famous astronaut is thinking is, "I was on the moon!" People come up to him and try to talk to him and he just smiles and nods because all he can hear is his mind saying, "I was on the moon!"

Crossing an Ironman finish line is every bit as awesome as it is hyped up to be. You will not be disappointed. In fact, you might never come down from the runner's high. Unlike the hype that surrounds the purchase of a new car or that vacation of a lifetime, there is no sense of remorse or emptiness at the end of this accomplishment. If anything, finishing an Ironman has been undersold. Chances are you've actually underestimated just how incredible it is going to be.

When I first registered for the Ironman, it seemed surreal — like telling people I was planning a trip to the moon. It sounded strange even to my own ears. "I'm going to do an Ironman," I would hear myself say to family and friends, but I wasn't sure if I entirely believed myself.

Each of the three events alone is long and difficult. Therein lies the beauty and the appeal of the Ironman. Few people on Earth will ever, in the course of their lives, complete a 2.4-mile swim, a 112-mile bike ride, or run a marathon. Even when taken individually, each event is pretty amazing, something to be respected. But when these three events are combined into one event — back, to back, to back — the result is something of awe, something legends are made of. Because it is absolutely unbelievable and anyone who can do it — not win it, but just complete the monster of an event, is forever called an Ironman.

As I swam, as I biked and as I ran, I was actually glad that each event was as long as it was. Even if I had the power on race day to snap my fingers and shorten the distance, there is no way that I would have shortened any of the three events. The insane duration is the key to the worthiness of the event. Any shorter and it wouldn't be impressive. If it were shorter then people wouldn't get tattoos to show they had finished. As the old quote goes, "Nothing difficult is ever easy."

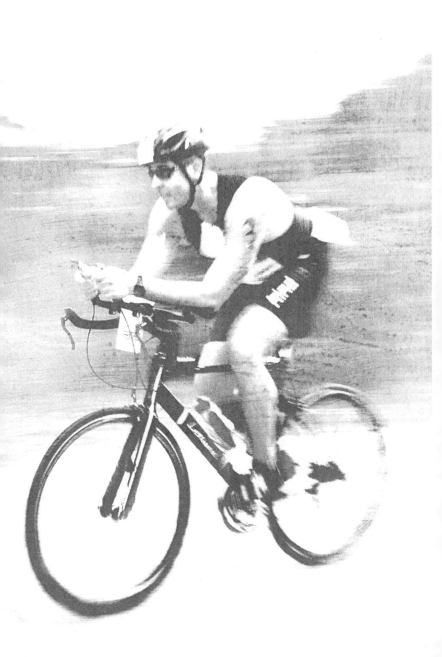

CHAPTER 5

THE EXCUSE

"People love to have lived a great story, but few people like the work it takes to make it happen." — Donald Miller

During the course of my training I learned through sweat, fatigue, muscle spasms and a little bit of blood that the human body is capable of extraordinary endurance if it is stretched just a little bit at a time. If you can ride your bike 10 miles and then jog half a mile this week, then you can certainly bike 11 miles and jog 3/4 of a mile next week. And so it is added and stretched just a little bit at a time. At first you barely swim one lap in the pool, then two, then three. At first it nearly kills you to bike 20 miles. Then you go for 25. Through first-hand lessons I learned a fact that few people would dare to believe. And that is, if a person is physically capable of swimming 10 meters, biking around the neighborhood and running across their yard then they *could* do an Ironman. Period.

The reason people do not want to believe this is because if they admit this to themselves then they are forced to confront the real reason why they "can't" do an Ironman — lack of determination. Ouch, that hurts and nobody wants to admit to him or herself that they lack the will and discipline. So it becomes much more convenient to say that they simply cannot do it. They lack the genes, the joints, the lungs, the whatever.

Actually, the best reason to not do an Ironman is that it is insane. I cannot argue with that. When folks say, "That's crazy! Why would I ever want to do an Ironman?" I can't argue with them. After all, it *is* crazy. But the one thing that I don't want to hear is, "Oh, I could never do an Ironman." Really? Tell that to the blind guy that did one in Louisville in 2009. Explain why it is that you cannot do an Ironman to the disabled people who cross the finish line in wheelchairs, or to the 70-year-old women that are Ironmen. So if you don't want to do an Ironman, fine. Just don't pretend that you don't have the ability.

The attribute that separates those who complete an Ironman from those who don't is not physical ability or gifts of superhuman endurance, but rather a plain and simple determination. Stubbornness is the one quality that all Ironmen share. All that it takes is an attitude that says, "I *will* do this." Whether it's raining, or cold, or you're changing your third flat tire, or maybe you're lucky enough to be dealing with all three, it takes a certain amount of what I call "stick-to-it-ness" to train for an Ironman.

No one will ever fault you for not doing an Ironman. You are perfectly within your right to say that it is crazy. You're right. And I can't blame you if decide not to try. But beware — that haunting question, "Could I do that?" will not go away. The Ironman World Championship will be televised every year, and every year you'll be reminded that tens of thousands of people from around the world became Ironmen that year. They went for it, they succeeded and they are just like you.

Anytime I've ever been faced with the dilemma between remaining comfortable or choosing to try something that might prove to be too difficult for me I always think of Theodore Roosevelt's famous speech "Citizenship In A Republic," delivered at the Sorbonne, in Paris, France on April 23, 1910. I memorized this when I was competing in Judo in college:

> *It is not the critic who counts: not the man who points out how the strong man stumbles or where the doer of deeds could have done better. The credit belongs to the man who is actually in the arena, whose face is marred by dust and sweat and blood, who strives valiantly, who errs and comes up short again and again, because there is no effort without error or shortcoming, but who knows the great enthusiasms, the great devotions, who spends himself for a worthy cause; who, at the best, knows, in the end, the triumph of high achievement, and who, at the worst, if he fails, at least he fails while daring greatly, so that his place shall never be with those cold and timid souls who knew neither victory nor defeat.*

I know that I'd rather fail while daring greatly than live the rest of my life not ever knowing if I had what it takes. If you're anything like me, you need to answer that question. You need to find out for sure. Chances are you're going to surprise yourself big time. You probably have no idea what your body is actually capable of. I know I didn't.

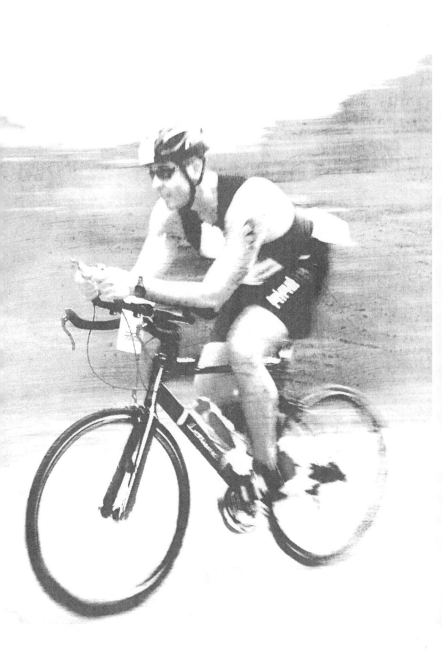

CHAPTER 6

THE CALLING

"Don't ask what the world needs. Ask what makes you come alive, and go do that. Because what the world needs is people who have come alive."
— Howard Thurman, speaking to Gil Bailie

Some people look out across a beautiful glassy lake and they want to paint a picture of it. Some people want to write a poem or sing a song about its beauty. Others may want to design a bridge that spans across it. I always want to see if I can swim to the other side of it.

I believe that this desire, this pull that we all have towards a different form of expression is a desire that was put there by God. Each of us bares a unique fingerprint that God placed on our hearts when he formed us in our mother's womb.

It is this calling that pulls us each towards different interests. Some people want to become doctors and some 3rd-grade teachers. Our Creator places these callings within each of us, and whether you call it a passion or a calling or a pull or attraction, there is something in each of us that yearns.

I once asked my wife Kerry to finish the sentence, "I feel most alive when I …" Kerry thought about it for a few seconds and then said, "When I take a photograph." This makes perfect sense. Kerry is a photographer. She has something in her that desires to take photos. I do not. I thought about the same question and answered, "When I'm running in the rain."

God calls each of us to do something great. Men have climbed Everest. Men have sailed around the world. Men have walked to the South Pole. All of these are different callings. There is a draw — an almost magnetic pull inside of us all toward something big.

To deny the calling within you is not simply depriving yourself of a richer and more meaningful life. It deprives all of mankind. The world only functions when everyone plays the part that was written for them. Imagine a world in which Roger Banister believed it impossible to break a four-minute mile, or one where Edmund Hillary was too busy with work to climb Everest. The world is a more beautiful place because Leonardo Da Vinci desired to paint the Mona Lisa, Gustave Eiffel engineered a tower, and because Julie Moss crawled across the finish line.

When human beings respond to the calling that God placed in their hearts, they enjoy something wonderful that not every human gets to feel. It is an amazing thing to be doing exactly what you yearn to do.

In *A Million Miles in a Thousand Years* — one of the best books I've ever read — Donald Miller writes, "If you watched a movie about a guy who wanted a Volvo and worked for years to get it, you wouldn't cry at the end when he drove off the lot, testing the windshield wipers ... But we spend years actually living those stories, and expect our lives to feel meaningful. The truth is, if what we choose to do with our lives won't make a story meaningful, it won't make a life meaningful either."

We are all writing the story of our lives. Every day, we write another piece of the legacy that we will leave behind. What will our kids and our grandkids say about us after we're gone? Will they say, "Boy, that Dave sure was punctual; and he had good penmanship." Or will they say things like, "My dad was an Ironman finisher." Or "My grandpa once swam two miles, biked 112 miles and then ran a marathon!"

Will the story of your life be worth telling? It will be for all of us if we dare to listen to that calling God put in our hearts. This might mean taking that first step and registering for the race that scares you more than any other race.

The first giant and frightening plunge you'll take into this Ironman adventure is to actually register for the event. This moment of registering, of clicking "Submit" on your online application, is almost as terrifying as the morning of the race itself. This is the commitment, the point of no return. This is when you make the decision to go all in.

I resisted the idea of registering for such a race. It was my good friend Lance who talked me into this endeavor in the first place. He was relentless. I explained countless times that this was not a good time in my life to bite off such a ludicrous venture. My job was crushing me as the operations scheduler in an Air Force flying squadron stationed in Okinawa. I worked nights, weekends and holidays. I regularly showed up to work at 2 or 3 a.m. It was crazy. Plus, I had two kids that I loved to spend time with, not to mention a couple of graduate classes in the evenings. Lance didn't care though. He was a single guy trying to keep his married friend from turning soft, and he was pretty good at it. Relentless might be a better word. After all, he is a salesman, and after several weeks I had decided he was right — we're not getting any younger and there will never be a convenient time to train.

Perhaps my ideal scenario was that the race was already filled up. Oh darn. Now I could say, "Yeah, I tried to register for an Ironman, but it was filled up. I'll try again next year." I'd get full credit for trying to register, but I'd get off the hook. As I clicked "Submit," part of me hoped that my computer would instantly get attacked by a virus or explode or that some other act of God would miraculously prevent me from actually getting accepted.

But then I got the email saying, "Congratulations on your acceptance into the Ironman." A part of me thought they were being sarcastic when they said congratulations.

Now I'd really done it. There was no going back. I was now $500 deep into this thing (registrations are expensive for races with this high level of support), and immediately my phone rang. It was my wife Kerry. She just called to say that she'd been doing some thinking and thought that this was really not a good time in our lives to attempt an Ironman. After all, she reasoned, the race is in Louisville, and we lived in Japan (some people get hung up on those sort of details). Kerry wanted me to wait a couple years when we'd be back in the States. I'd be done with my grad school and it would all make sense. It would be much more practical then.

"I really wish you would have called about two minutes ago," I said.

She sighed.

"But don't worry," I said, "I'm looking at some inexpensive bikes online."

Another sigh.

I suggested we meet for lunch at her favorite restaurant. I knew I had to dig my way out of the hole I'd gotten into.

The moment you decide to register is the moment you decide to start living out the story that was written for your character. Once you make that decision, click "Submit," and plunge into your Ironman, your life will change. It's like pulling down the lap bar on a roller coaster and feeling it click. And this ride will last for one year.

You're not even sure if it's a smart decision (you see the lake). It's a lot of money (you're standing on the shore). But it's a whole year away (you're thinking about it). It would be awesome to do (you're running down the dock). It would feel incredible to finish an Ironman (cannonball). Click "Submit" (splash).

Whatever your calling is, whatever it is that you feel a yearning to do, you either need to start painting the lake or jump into it.

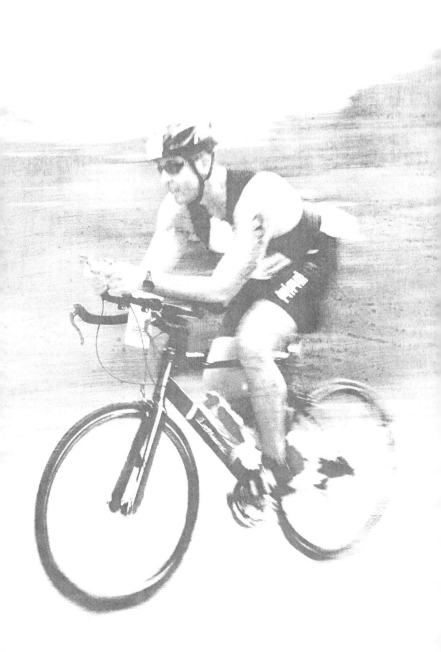

CHAPTER 7

THE EVERYMAN

*"The greatest works are done by the ones. The hundreds do not often
do much, the companies never; it is the units, the single individuals,
that are the power and the might" — Charles Spurgeon*

Ironman has been referred to as "Everyman's
Everest" and I think that is a pretty good analogy. It's the
biggest mountain that I'll probably ever climb. It appears
insurmountable at first glance, but the more you train and the
closer you get to it the more you begin to realize that it's just
a matter of climbing one inch at a time. It's just a mountain
and you just put one foot in front of the other. I remember
the pre-race briefing given to all the athletes the night before
the Ironman. There was a speaker who gave us a lecture on
the rules, and another who spoke about safety and logistical
concerns. The final speaker was to explain the nuances of the
event — specifically the run. He cleared his throat, paused for
a second and then said, "Left foot, right foot, left foot, repeat.
Any questions?" And that was it.

For all of the complexities of training and the
carbon fiber bikes and the hydrodynamic swim skins available
on the market, it really all comes down to putting one foot in
front of the other, continuing to move forward one inch at a
time, no matter what. The race official, on the morning of the
race announced, "You can't control the hills or the weather

or flat tires or getting kicked in the face by the swimmer in front of you. There is only one thing that you have any control over at all, and that's your attitude. So enjoy your race day and keep a good attitude no matter what gets thrown at you." That was pretty good advice for the race; it was pretty good advice for life actually.

One of the most instantly confronting sights at any Ironman race is that everyone in it looks…well, normal. If you've never before watched an Ironman event in person, then you might have some preconceived notions and stereotypes about what the athletes look like. Your stereotype has most likely been influenced by the media, by magazine covers and by underwear ads on billboards. You've been shown in large, glossy, re-touched photos your entire life what a "fit" person looks like. You've been sold on the "Abs Special Edition" of Men's Health and so you think you know a fit person when you see one.

Then you witness an Ironman. Here you'll see average looking folks from all walks of life. It really looks like a complete random sampling of folks from your local YMCA. True, you won't see any 400-pound people, but you're not going to see a lot of underwear models with 6-pack abs either. Why? Because that Calvin Klein guy that you think represents "fitness" actually just represents 1,000 crunches a day and no carbs. But these stereotyped physiques don't have any practical application. They're like vehicles that were designed exclusively for car shows. Get them on the racetrack (or heaven forbid off-road) and you'd quickly see what they're really made of.

The real Ironman, however, looks just like you and me. I saw folks who were carrying around a few extra pounds and several extra years pass right by me. They were extremely friendly as they passed, but I wouldn't want to try to stand in their way. Because the one feature that is shared by all the athletes is not external at all — it's not 3 percent body fat and it's certainly not chiseled abs. It is the fierce determination that they will not quit. They will keep going no matter how tough it gets. Not tough as in "my agent did not have my soy latte ready, and the magazine photographer is talking snooty to me." But tough as in, "I stopped being able to feel my legs at mile 80 of the bike, and at mile 18 of the run I noticed my socks were covered in blood." That's the kind of athlete you'll find at an Ironman — an average looking person with love handles, a goofy swimsuit and a determination that you can see in the eyes.

Chances are, you will not ever play in the NFL. You probably won't get called up to the major league, and no matter how much you shoot hoops in your driveway, it's not going to get you into the NBA. But the odds of you becoming an Ironman are actually very good. This is one sporting event you have a shot at. It requires no unique, one-in-a-million-like talent. People of all ages, all handicaps and all conditions have succeeded. The only thing you need is determination.

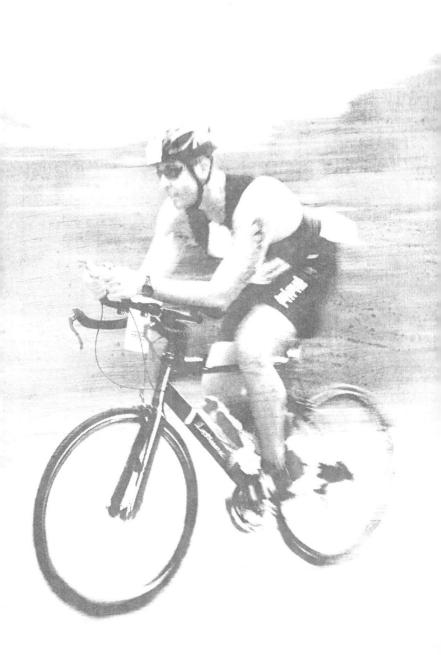

{ CHAPTER 8 }

THE FAMILY

"A good example has twice the value of good advice"
— Unknown

You know that scene in Rocky IV — the training montage — where Rocky is training in snowy Russia? That's what it feels like to be an Average Joe training for an Ironman Triathlon. You've got your professional triathletes — your Dolph Lundgrens — and they have fancy indoor trainers, power meters on their bikes and carbon fiber sunglasses that match their Speedo. And there you are biking uphill pulling your kids behind you in a trailer. While the kids eat snacks and read books, your legs are cranking with everything you've got. You go for training runs pushing your kid in a jogging stroller. You sprint up hills giving piggyback rides. Like Rocky pulling a sled through the snow with Pauly in it, or lifting an oxcart with his family inside. You're like Rocky — no frills, no expensive gadgets. It doesn't require a staff of professional trainers or a gym membership. All you really need is heart. You swim a lot, bike a lot and run a lot. It's really that simple.

So incorporate your family in your workouts. Whether on your back, behind your bike, or being pushed or pulled along. Small kids will love it. It's bonding, and it will break up the monotony of your workouts. Hey, if it worked for

Rocky, then it's got to be good.

Kids love to help with even the littlest things. They want to help pump up your bike tires and fill water bottles. Give them someone to cheer for. Be their superhero. If nothing else, you'll teach them how to reach their goals. You'll demonstrate for them to never give up. You will embody dedication. For the rest of their lives they will carry that lesson with them. "My Dad is an Ironman." "My Mom is an Ironman." Like going back to school to finish a degree, accomplishing an Ironman is a legacy for the whole family to be proud of. They will share in your accomplishment and recognize the new height to which you have set the bar for them. You'll teach them to dream big!

My son Luke was begging to go for a run with me as I laced up my shoes and filled my pockets with Goo packs. "Dad, please let me run with you! I can run really far! I won't slow you down, I promise!" How do you say no to that? I tried to no avail to explain how far 13 miles was. I even attempted a lame analogy with my arms, explaining that, "Daddy is going to run this much!" stretching my arms out wide. His eyes were just gazing up at me as if I'd just read a chapter from the U.S. tax code. "Alright!" I relented. "You can run with me. Yes, of course little Braeden can run too." I had opened the floodgates.

We have gone over this routine countless times since that day. Saying yes to them and including them in my run that day was a priceless move. The way it works is I jog with them for as long as they can go. I encourage them to "run to just one more mailbox," or "just up one more hill, come on, you can do it!" Then I jog back home with them, leave them with a high-five and continue on with my run alone. This only costs me about five to 10 minutes, but it is usually the highlight of my day.

As Luke got stronger he could ride his bike along with me while I ran. This worked out great for both of us. He's reveling in the fact that he's beating me — never mind the fact that he's on a bike — he's just happy he's faster than his dad!

There is a notorious trail in Okinawa, Japan, known as the Habu Trail. It is a windy and very hilly paved trail through the jungle. It was my favorite place to run on the island. Eventually, I worked out a deal with Luke that if he could ride his bike the entire length of the trail with me, making it up every hill on his own, then I would buy him the Camelback water pack he had been wanting. One hot day we were both laboring up the last big hill, me jogging, and Luke riding his little red bike. He didn't quite make it and he was forced off his bike. In tears, he pushed his bike the rest of the way up the hill. He was devastated thinking he'd lost the Camelback. But I was all smiles and cheers. I explained to him that he had made it up every hill on his own. I didn't care if he rode his bike, pushed it, or carried it on his head. I was just proud that he didn't quit. We enjoyed the Habu trail many times together after that, and with his water supply on his back, the hills seemed to get a littler easier for him every time.

If you want your kids to live healthy lives, to put down the chips and the video games, then what better way than to set the example yourself. And what better example than to become an Ironman? When a child sees his parent turn off the TV, stop buying ice cream and start a regular workout routine, that kid learns first hand how to make healthy choices in life.

Of course, I was not always the perfect model of the parent-triathlete combination. I had my uglier moments to be sure. There were times when I just couldn't even seem to get my socks on without kids crawling all over me. If I'm reaching for my shoes then suddenly my kids become interested in trying them on first and running around the house in them. They might not ever notice or care about my cycling gloves, but they suddenly find the need to wear them when they see me pick them up.

With my visor and sunglasses on, sunscreen applied, iPod playlist ready to go and water bottle in hand, Kerry must have sensed that I had one foot out the door as she called down, "Hey Babe, I need you to change Braeden's diaper for me! I'm busy with Luke."

"Uh, sure, Honey!" I replied. Sunglasses off, ear buds removed, water bottle down.

I wish I could tell you this only happened once. But if you've got kids and you're considering an Ironman — just go ahead and accept your fate.

As adults, we are always telling our kids that they can do anything they put their mind to. We teach them to dream big, to reach for the stars. We tell them they can be anything they want to be when they grow up and that if they work hard enough anything is possible. Prove it to them. Show them that you're not just feeding them fairy tales when you say that they can do the impossible. It will be a lesson they never forget, and will be a legacy they pass on to their children one day.

For Christians like me, this is also a perfect teaching opportunity to illustrate Philippians 4:13, which says, "I can do all things through Christ who strengthens me." What better way to demonstrate the truth of this verse and the power of God to your children? Your entire training experience will become a metaphor for this verse.

While we're on the subject, I also made the decision to illustrate to my kids that Ironman training was not going to take priority over church. Now I'm not saying that I've got the world's most perfect attendance record, but I knew it would be wrong for my wife and kids to go to church while dad got to ride his bike. So I forfeited what seemed to always be the most perfect training weather (as luck would have it) and take my family to church every Sunday morning. Then I would start my training after lunch.

Besides, how could I pray for God to help me and bless my efforts or to keep me safe on the road when I'm blowing off worshipping him in order to train? I wanted to make God a part of my training. So when you're already working your training schedule around work and ball games and kid's piano lessons, surely you can work it around two hours of church.

A key part of Ironman training is doing what is known in the triathlon world as a "brick." A brick is when you do one event immediately after another one. Like going for a bike ride then going for a run, or going for a swim and then going for a bike ride. Bricks are essential to training for your Ironman because they get your legs used to the idea of running after biking or biking after swimming. This type of muscle and joint familiarity will pay dividends during your race; you wouldn't want your first ever bike-run combo to be on the big day. So doing a bike-run brick became a regular weekend activity for me.

For this reason, I always viewed playing with my sons Luke and Braeden as part of my training. Being Dad was just another part of my brick. I couldn't spend the rest of the day after a long bike ride sacked out on the couch — not if I expected to run a marathon after biking 112 miles. So I made up my mind to mount my bike or go for my long run early in the day, then instead of resting afterwards I would take my boys swimming, to a park or just wrestle with them in the living room. So my bricks became bike-run-play.

My longest training day ever was the Saturday that I biked 96 miles, then immediately showered and drove my kids two hours north for a half-day trip to the Ocean Expo Park. This forced me to view the bike ride as no big deal. It was just an insignificant early morning workout — nothing more. I was not going to make a big deal of riding for six hours by spending the remainder of the day resting.

I always had this mantra running through the back of my mind: "And you plan on running a marathon after biking 112 miles?" This little voice of skepticism in the back of my mind kept me from complaining or seeking sympathy after my training rides.

Dean Karnazes illustrates this point so perfectly in his amazing book *Ultramarathoner: Confessions of an All-night Runner*, when he describes completing a 200-mile run and then going to an amusement park with his kids. Contrary to assumption, my experience is that training for an ultra-endurance event brings families closer. A dad who can find

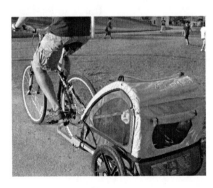

{ *Taking my son for a bike work-out with me helped keep the kids involved in my training.* }

the time and energy to train for an Ironman is usually the kind of dad who can find time for his kids, and he'll have the energy or at least training mentality to be able to play with them, too. It seems to be the sedentary, lazy men who can't seem to find the time or energy for anything other than watching television with their kids.

My best training day ever on the road to my Ironman was the day I was doing my last long bike ride — an 80 miler. I was battling a brutal head wind, on a long uphill, and lost in my own thoughts when I felt a vehicle slowing down behind me and then I heard it honk. There in the family minivan was my wife and two boys cheering me on and clapping for me. Suddenly I felt like I had just turned onto the Champs-Élysées in the final stage of the Tour de France. They handed me a peanut butter and banana sandwich (the perfect endurance nutrition, by the way) and passed me several new bottles of cold Gatorade out the car window in exchange for my empty ones. As they drove away I was completely recharged and my spirit had been renewed. I had been awakened from the drudgery of my training ride and was reminded of why I was doing this training and just how awesome that finish line in Louisville was going to feel.

{ TIP: MAKE SURE YOU HAVE YOUR BIKE FITTED TO YOU BY A PRO AT YOUR LOCAL BIKE SHOP. THE INCREASE IN COMFORT, EFFICIENCY AND POWER ARE PRICELESS. IT CAN ALSO PREVENT INJURIES. }

Throughout my training, my kids drew me pictures

and made signs and banners to encourage me. They were awesome! There is still a crayon-drawn Ironman symbol taped to the inside of our front door. It was there to greet me when I returned from having completed my 140.6 miles in Louisville and I don't think I'll ever be able to take it down.

A big piece of training advice that I would give to any family man or woman seeking to do an Ironman would be to tell your spouse what you need from them. Communication is going to be even more crucial than ever during your training. Marriage is hard enough without one of you trying to torture yourself on a bicycle every weekend. Tell your spouse that you need encouragement or that you could use some motivation in certain areas. Don't expect them to read your mind or even be on the same page as you. They've probably never been in this situation before either.

In fact, this endeavor of yours is a big deal for them as well. Now that you're out there burning up the road, they are probably doing more than ever in terms of taking care of the kids, cleaning the house and cooking meals. Make sure you put as much effort into your family as you do your training. Now that the quantity of time you get to spend with them on weekends is going to be decreased by several hours, make sure that you increase the quality of the time. And remember that this is only for one season of life. The training is temporary but the accomplishment will last you forever.

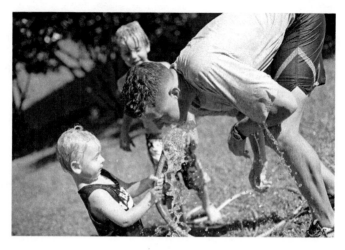

{ *Enjoying a post-run cool down in the backyard with my boys. This gave everybody something to look forward to at the end of daddy's run!* }

At the time I was training for the Ironman, my wife was starting her business as an on-location photographer. That meant that people hired her to come take their family photos at their favorite park or in their own yard or at the beach. So as I tried to plan out my weekend training run or ride I would have to wheel and deal with Kerry as to when she would watch the kids for me and when I would watch the kids for her. The logic usually went like this: if it was raining then she could not do a photo shoot, therefore that would be the perfect time for me to train. But if the weather was perfect and sunny, then I would have to watch the kids so she could go take photos. It was a marvelous Catch-22 that I could not argue my way out of and it resulted in me getting very comfortable running and biking in the rain. So much so that it felt strangely out of place to run in dry socks and shoes.

Remember, you only get one chance to do your first Ironman. So make it a great experience for the entire family. Let your kids fill your water bottles and tell them you couldn't have finished the bike ride without their help. Make the Ironman a family affair.

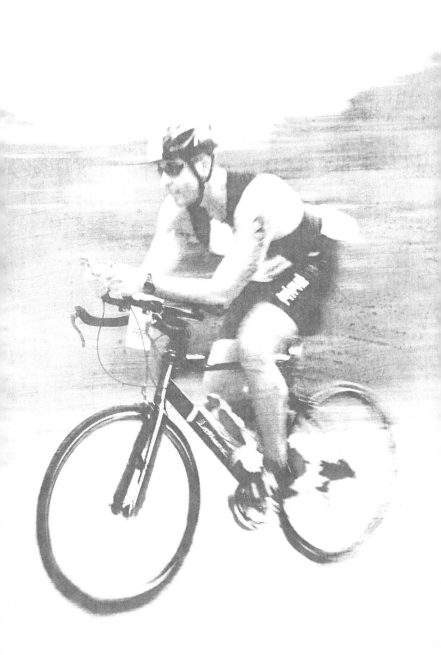

CHAPTER 9

THE JOB

"Opportunity is missed by most people because it is dressed in overalls and looks like work." — *Thomas A. Edison*

Your job. It's maybe the biggest single obstacle in your way of training for an Ironman. Let's face it; you don't own your own schedule. There were so many sunny, 70-degree days with not a cloud in the sky that I had to spend in my windowless office staring at a computer screen or making phone calls to folks who had no idea the training opportunity I was forfeiting for the sake of that conversation.

Just in case you're thinking that your job is more demanding than mine, or that I could not possibly understand your unique circumstances, just in case you're thinking the hours you work make it impossible for you to train for such a demanding triathlon, let me assure you — it can be done.

The Guinness Book of World Records has not yet officially declared it, but working for the 82d Reconnaissance Squadron at Kadena Air Base, Japan, might just be the craziest hours a human can work. As a mission director, operations scheduler and navigator, my job kept me coming in at all hours of the day, the night, the weekends and especially the holidays. I came in to work every single Saturday for my first year on the job, and I remember once going for three months without a weekend off. That's just the way it had to be. It was business as usual, and we all carried the load with only minor grumbling.

So this was the atmosphere in which I carved out my training plan. There were many days when I had to work out before going to work. These were the days when I could anticipate a 12-14 hour workday. I knew I'd have to eat lunch at my desk and I could see ahead of time that I would not have the energy or motivation to work out when my workday ended late at night. So on days like this I'd have to go for an early morning run or 5 a.m. swim.

Other times I would have to go in to work at 1 or 2 a.m. There was no way to work out before work in that situation. I would only be getting two or three hours of sleep anyway. So on these days — which were definitely the most painful — I would usually work out after my shift ended. This usually meant being sleep deprived and in a zombie-like state even though it was only 2 p.m. But if it was sunny outside I could fool my body into waking back up. Sometimes though, I just needed a nap first. This usually turned out to be a big mistake. I would wake up from these naps feeling worse than before; I wouldn't even be sure what day it was. My wife could tell you stories about the phone ringing during my nap, and me, thinking that the sound was from my alarm clock, would instinctively jump right into the shower.

The best days were of course the normal ones when you come to work at 7:30 a.m. and you leave about eight or nine hours later. I learned to appreciate these rare workdays that so many people take for granted.

So because of those ever-changing work schedules, I could never really get in a routine with my workouts. I had to take it one day at a time, and always keep my workout times flexible.

On one particularly beautiful day, I packed a gym bag with my swim gear in it and planned for a swim workout during my lunch break, only to discover after arriving at work that there would be no lunch break for me that day and that I would be busy until late that night. Of course the sunny weather had given way to rain by that night, and my swim workout had to be changed to a run.

Business trips are the other major obstacle that your job will throw at you. In the Air Force, they call these trips TDYs (short for Temporary Duty), and I definitely had enough TDYs to keep me distracted from my training.

My best advice here is to just maintain the fitness level that you've got while you're on a business trip. This probably won't be the time or place to set any new personal records or push yourself for a longer distance than you've ever done before. But try not to slide backwards either. Make it your goal to just do something.

While living in Japan, I had a one-week trip to San Antonio, Texas right in the middle of my training. Being completely jet-lagged and unable to sleep, I found the hotel fitness room at about 3 a.m. and ran one of best nine-mile runs on a treadmill ever. Those are the kinds of workouts you'll never forget.

I found a treadmill to run on every time I went TDY. I ran along the beach while I was in Guam. I swam laps in an indoor pool in Omaha. I ran outside in Virginia. In Tokyo, I rode a stationary bike for an hour then ran on a treadmill for 30 minutes.

Business trips are also difficult because you're eating out a lot. I wish I could tell you that I ordered grilled chicken and bought fresh fruit. But the truth is I love food. I splurged right along with the rest of my crew (what can I say, I'm an Average Joe). But I got up the next morning and at least tried to sweat off as much as I could.

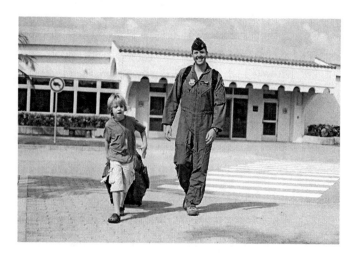

{ *Coming back home from one of my many "business trips."* }

The most important things to remember about balancing work with training are to be flexible with your workout plan and remain consistent when you're on the road.

Think of your workouts as deposits into a retirement account. There's no one huge deposit that is going to make you retire in comfort. It's simply the culmination of all those little deposits that you made over time. The same thing is true for training. Don't expect one humongous workout to make you ready for an Ironman. But you do have to be consistent with your deposits. So when work throws crazy hours or business trips your way, just relax and accept that you might need to adjust your workouts a little bit. Just as long as you're depositing something into your account, you're still moving in the right direction.

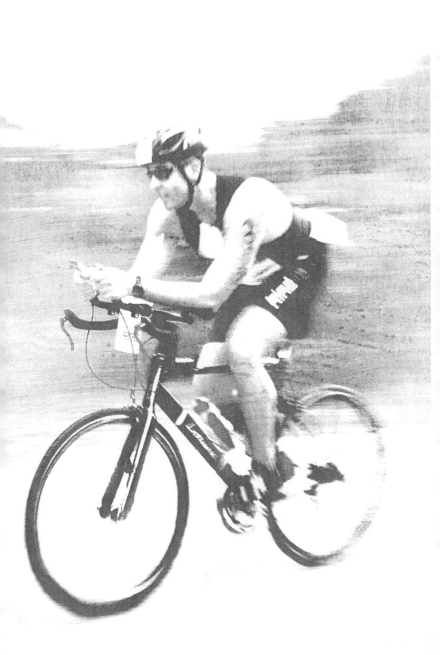

CHAPTER 10

THE SWIM

"No man drowns if he perseveres in praying to God, and can swim."
— Russian Proverb

Do you know why I love the swim so much? Because it's like the cover charge to get into the Ironman race. The very idea of swimming 2.4 miles is what keeps many potential racers from even registering. It's intimidating. I've heard people say, "I could probably bike 112 miles if I had to, and I've run a marathon before, but there is no way I could swim 2.4 miles." The swim portion is like the bouncer at the door and if you want to make it to the party inside you've got to train and find a way to overcome your fear in order to get past that beast of a swim. The swim portion keeps out the riff-raff.

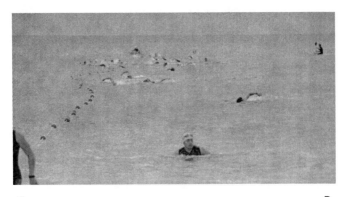

{ *The Torii Station Sprint Triathlon in Okinawa, Japan. The East China Sea was rough that day. (I'm the one on the right with my left arm in the air.)* }

As I mentioned before, most of the swimming that I did in training was done during weekday lunch breaks. I would go to the fitness center and swim laps for about 45 minutes to an hour.

Now I've never been on a swim team before. I've never been a member of a Masters swim group. I don't do "sets," and I don't count meters. I wasn't training to become a swimmer; I was training to become an Ironman. So all that mattered to me was being able to swim freestyle a very long way — 2.4 miles to be exact.

When I was in college I decided to try lap swimming as a workout. I was in descent shape from playing soccer. But when I first got in the pool I was truly humbled. After huffing and puffing and splashing and choking with all the strength and energy that I had in me, I had swam two laps (four lengths) of the pool. I still remember it like it was yesterday. There was a big fat man in the lane beside of me and he was swimming laps so effortlessly. He was swimming laps when I got there and he was still swimming laps when I left. What the heck was going on? I was in shape, I was young, I was strong — why couldn't I swim more? This question frustrated and upset me.

I swam a lot that summer before my sophomore year of college. By the end of the summer it had clicked. I had learned that swimming was not about raw strength or force, and the type of fitness it required was vastly different from the fitness required to run or play soccer. Swimming was about technique, it was about being able to relax, it was about being smooth. Like learning to ride a bike for the first time — eventually it just clicks. I finally figured out how to exhale under the water then turn my head to the side to breathe. I finally figured out how often I needed that breath of air, so I developed a rhythm to turn my head and breathe on every third arm strong. I was finally relaxed in the water. Eventually it wasn't really like a workout any more as long as I went slow enough. By the end of the summer I could swim one mile without ever stopping.

So when I decided 11 years after that to train for an Ironman, I was able to recall my technique for swimming. Go slow. Stay relaxed. Now 2.4 miles is about 80 laps in a 25-meter pool. That's 160 lengths. That's a long way to swim. That's a long time to be immersed in water even if you're not swimming.

{ TIP: IF YOU'RE AFRAID OF HAVING YOUR GOGGLES KICKED OFF OF YOUR FACE BY THE SWIMMER IN FRONT OF YOU THEN PUT ON YOUR GOGGLES FIRST, THEN YOUR SWIM CAP. THE CAP WILL HOLD THEM IN PLACE EVEN IF THEY GET KICKED. }

And it's really a long time to wear goggles that are trying to suck your eyeballs right out of your head.

So my goal for training for the Ironman swim was (much like my goal for the bike and run) just finish the thing before the cutoff time, and conserve as much energy as possible for the next event. In the water, it's all about energy conservation. You can't fight against the water. You can't beat it into submission. You have to become one with it. You have to slice your way through it. And most importantly you have to relax.

Swimming was the only one of the three disciplines that actually left me feeling energized. Biking and running exhausted me. But a nice relaxed swim in chilly water on a cool morning was refreshing. Unfortunately for me, those cool mornings came to a screeching halt in Okinawa

{ **TIP: DON'T USE TINTED SWIM GOGGLES. THE SUN WILL BARELY EVEN BE OUT, AND IT WILL PROBABLY BE PLENTY DARK ALREADY.** }

around April. The Ironman I was training for was at the end of August and for the five months leading up to the race I was swimming in about 90-degree temperature (lunch break = high noon) with the sun beating down on me and the water felt like it was just a few degrees shy of boiling.

When I wasn't swimming on a lunch break I might wake up around 4:30 in the morning and jog to the pool, swim for an hour and then jog back home for my shower and coffee.

This was my exact routine on the one and only time that I swam the full 2.4 miles during training. I wanted to do it at least once. It would eliminate another unknown from race day. I was curious to see how close I would be to the two hours and 20 minutes cutoff time. I arrived at the pool when it opened at 5 a.m., slightly winded from the jog there. I ran there in the new tri suit that had just arrived in the mail, because I knew that you were supposed to test everything in training — nothing new should be tried for the first time on race day. I took off my running shoes and jumped in the pool.

When I got out of the pool after one hour and 40 minutes of non-stop freestyle swimming, the lifeguard got out of his chair, approached me and asked, "Dude, how far did you just swim?"

"Eighty laps," I said. The sun was just coming up. I smiled as I jogged back home. I knew I could make the time cutoff. And having been a lifeguard myself in college (following that summer of learning to swim laps) I knew that it takes a heck of a long swim to impress a lifeguard.

My first swim in a triathlon was in a really short sprint triathlon in San Antonio, Texas. It was 2003 and I was a second lieutenant in the Air Force attending navigator training at Randolph Air Force Base.

I'm not really sure what made me enter this race but I was always intentionally doing things that violated my comfort zone. If the thought of something made me uneasy or even better if it outright scared me then I would have to make myself do it. Sort of a sick twisted game of psychology that I guess I've always played. But anyway, the swim for my very first tri was in an outdoor pool. It was something like a 400-meter swim, 16-mile bike and a 3-mile run. Something close to that.

Everyone was lined up in a gigantic single file line and we entered the pool one at a time with a few seconds separating us. Our timing chip we wore on our ankle would start our race time as we entered the pool. I remember being so excited and nervous and having so much adrenaline pumping as I got closer and closer to the front of the line. When it came my turn and I dove in, I felt fantastic; I was swimming my best ever. I had never gone that fast before. Then I suddenly realized why. I was not breathing. I did about 40 meters without ever turning my head to breathe. I had just kept my head under water and swam as fast as I could. But when my brain finally realized my body's stupid plan it sent an S.O.S. out to BREATHE IMMEDIATELY! I then lost all prior smoothness by having to swim the next lap with my head entirely out of the water sucking in as much oxygen as possible. I finally got settled back down and finished the last few laps in my standard rhythm.

Contrast this over-eagerness to go fast and not breathe with what I saw at the Wisconsin Ironman in 2006. When the cannon went off and the 2,000 people started swimming, I noticed a group of about two dozen individuals that were out in the water but they weren't swimming. They were stretching. They were talking. They were putting on their goggles and adjusting their swim caps. "What are you thinking! The race has started! Did you not hear the massive cannon?!" My mind was amazed by the leisurely calm of these swimmers. Then one by one they each started the swim. These nameless, faceless individuals out there in the water would later become my role models for Ironman training.

I didn't understand these folks or their lackadaisical attitude until I started training for my own Ironman; and then everything they did made sense. It was the Tortoise vs. The Hare. They understood that it wasn't about going fast and it wasn't about shaving a few seconds or even minutes off their time. Ironman is not a sprint. Heck, it's not even a marathon (though there will be one of those included later in the day). Ironman is an all-day-dig-down-deep-ultra-endurance event that will test your religion, your faith in mankind and your mind's ability to hold down a sports

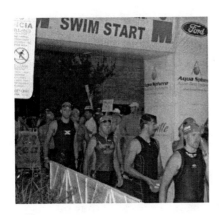

Getting ready to jump into the Ohio River at the start of the 2009 Louisville Ironman. The sun was just coming up and we were all nervous. (I'm in the one still holding my swim cap)

drink when your stomach wants so badly to throw it up.

Now if you've never gone for a swim before with several thousand of your closest friends, an Ironman swim can be a little intimidating. It has best been described as being in a washing machine full of arms and legs. I found that to be pretty accurate. There will be hands clawing at your feet and ankles and you'll think they're trying to drown you or at least rip off your timing chip. There will be feet kicking you in the head. You won't be able to see them but you'll swim right into them. And there will always be that one jerk doing a breaststroke and you will really not see it coming when he kicks you in the head. I've seen goggles broken or lost, a few bloody noses and one nose that was completely broken and the individual dropped out in order to seek medical help. Those are the few and far between extreme cases though. Most of us just get a few friendly kicks in the face, a few claws to the ankles and one person who actually swims right over the top of us. That's right. On land you must go around a person in order to pass them. You have to go right or left. Not true in the water where there exists a third option.

So by now in my training I'm realizing that those swimmers that waited for the smoke to clear before they entered into the fray were really the smart ones.

I entered in an 88-kilometer tri in Japan with distances that were almost exactly a half-ironman. It was called the Izena 88, and it did wonders for boosting my self-confidence. It had a seven-hour cutoff and I thought, okay, if I can do this thing then I'll see about doing a full-distance triathalon next. The swim at the Izena 88 was the most picturesque swim imaginable. It was a beach start into the East China Sea and the water was absolutely brilliant. It was clear blue and perfectly calm. I lost track of time and distance during the swim. I was staring down at starfish and sea cucumbers and fish of every color. I even saw scuba divers down there who were watching us all from below. Before I knew it the swim was over and it was time to get on my bike.

{ TIP: HOLD OFF ON PUTTING SUNSCREEN ON YOUR UPPER ARMS OR CALFS UNTIL AFTER THE BODY MARKING ON RACE MORNING. THE MARKER WON'T WRITE ON YOUR SKIN IF IT'S COVERED IN SUNSCREEN. }

Never again would I enjoy such a scenic swim. My Ironman was in the Ohio River, and you could not see even two inches in front of you. I was swimming in a brown fog that obscured the guy in front completely until he kicked me in the head. In Louisville's defense, however, it was a scenic swim above the water. The city skyline was beautiful from the river and it was pretty cool swimming under all those bridges.

My best advice for the swim is to get yourself into a comfortable rhythm that you can relax in. You should think of the swim as a stretching exercise before the rest of the day.

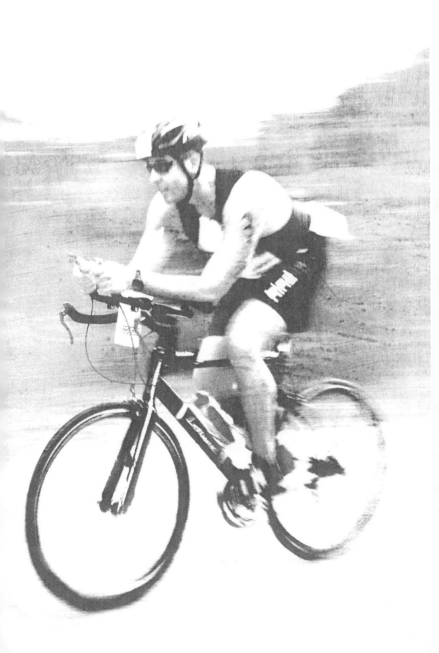

CHAPTER 11

THE BIKE

"I thought about that while riding my bike." — *Albert Einstein*

The hardest part for me on my road to becoming an Ironman was getting on my bike on those lazy Saturday mornings or those sleepy Sunday afternoons. Instead of laying on the couch watching football or going to see a movie I made myself go ride a bike for four, five, or six hours. I no longer thought of my training in terms of miles, but rather hours.

Here's what it was like on my typical weekend. I would cover myself in sunscreen, mix three bottles of Gatorade and mount them to my bike, make peanut butter bagels wrapped in plastic, put power bars and a banana in the pockets of my cycling jersey. I would put enough change in my zippered pocket for drink machines along the way to refill my water bottles. (I would easily drink 10 to 12 bottles of fluid during a five-hour bike ride on a 90-degree day, far more than can be carried on the bike at one time.) Next I would stuff my Bento Box (a very tiny "lunch box" that attaches to the upper tube of a bike) with as many goo packs as it could hold, spray some lube on my

{ TIP: BIKING WITHOUT AT LEAST TWO SPARE TUBES IS LIKE PLAYING RUSSIAN ROULETTE. }

chain, inflate the tires to 125 psi, reset the computer that tracked my speed, distance and pace, pack three spare tubes and two spare chain links, calculate the hours of daylight remaining, put an ibuprofen in a Ziploc bag along with a cell phone, put on my gloves, fasten my helmet, clip into my pedals and get settled into a comfortable position for the next 80 or so miles.

I bought my first road bike from a guy in San Antonio who had been renting bikes to tourists for decades. This bike had untold mileage on it and no telling how many riders had taken great care of it, the level of care that only a renter can provide. I paid 90 dollars for it and insisted that

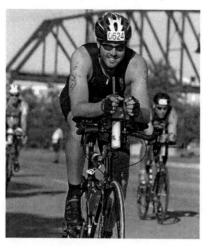

Right out of the water and just embarking on the 112 mile bike ride. I was euphoric just thinking about how the swim portion was now behind me.

he include a helmet with the purchase. I had just registered for my first tri and up until that point the only bikes I had ever ridden were my Huffy that my parents bought for me from a yard sale when I was about seven and the Mongoose mountain bike that I bought from Wal-Mart when I was in college. But now I had my first real road bike, with the skinny tires, drop down handlebars and 10 speeds. The best part: it was a Dave Scott Ironman bike made by Centurion, and had this tri I was racing in been in 1985 instead of 2003, then my bike would have made me look like a serious competitor. But after 18 years of trading paint for rust this bike was just one flat tire away from being totaled.

I wasn't very familiar with cycling in general. I had never worn shoes that clipped into pedals before. I had never changed a tube or a chain, and I was certainly not about to shave my legs or wear those ridiculous cycling shorts. (Note: After training for an Ironman, I became intimately familiar with all of those things ... except for the shaving part, because hey, if you're at the back of the pack do a few seconds really make much difference?)

Of the three events in triathlon, cycling is the most time consuming. You'll spend most of your training hours on the saddle of your bike. For that reason alone, I would consider it the most important of the three disciplines for anyone set on becoming an Ironman. A long swim is only an hour, a long run is only two or three hours, but a long bike ride is six hours or more. The bike is really the heart and soul of the Ironman. By the day's end you'll barely even remember that there was a swim earlier that morning, but there's nothing forgettable about biking 112 miles.

The bike is also the only part of the triathlon in which

you are dependent upon a machine. The swim is all about your arms and legs, the run is all about your legs, but the bike forces you to trust a couple of wheels and a chain. This fact was not lost on me. It made me paranoid to think that all of my training and all of my work I'd put into this race for over a year might all come crashing down if I wrecked my bike and damaged it bad enough. I also realized that for a guy who's aiming to finish pretty close to the time cutoff I wouldn't have a whole lot of time to spend fiddling around with flat tires.

{ TIP: USE CHEAP WATER BOTTLES IN YOUR BIKE ON RACE DAY, BECAUSE YOU'LL HAVE TO DISCARD THEM IN ORDER TO TAKE THE BOTTLES THEY HAND YOU ALONG THE RIDE. AND YOU'LL NEVER SEE THEM AGAIN. }

By now I had decided to upgrade from my '85 Centurion to a proper tri bike. Complete with aerobars and an aluminum and carbon frame, I would not be able to blame my bike if anything went wrong. I actually practiced changing flats, too. I looked forward to getting a flat on a training ride because it would give me a chance to time myself and practice. I never biked anywhere without two spare tubes and a patch kit.

Part of the spirit of Ironman is self-sufficiency. You can't accept any outside aid from friends or family, and no one else on a bike can lend you any tools or help either. If you're lucky enough to be in the vicinity of one of the official race support vans, then you might get some help — but you'd better not bank on that; 112 miles is a lot of road for that van to cover and there are going to be a lot of other folks out there with problems. The idea is to be able to handle whatever is thrown at you while on the course. Flat tire? Change it yourself. Broken chain? Should've carried a chain tool and a spare link. Bent wheel? Disconnect your brakes so it can still spin. Wrapped your bike around a tree? Throw it over your shoulder and start jogging earlier than you'd originally planned.

The farthest distance that I ever rode in training was 96 miles. It took me 6.5 hours to do it and that included stopping at the Japanese equivalent of a 7-Eleven for some rice balls wrapped in seaweed. The sun was tormenting me on this mammoth of a bike ride, and I was chugging liquids like never before. I finally pulled over at a roadside store and rewarded myself with this tasty Japanese snack and stretched my back and neck for a few moments of much-needed relief. It's called onigiri, and if you're ever biking through Okinawa I recommend stopping for a mid-ride snack at Family Mart. There's a peculiar satisfaction that creeps over you as you realize you are now going farther than you've ever gone before. You're entering uncharted territory.

I learned that a strong headwind is actually worse than riding up hill. You can see a definite end at the top of a hill and you strive towards that goal, but there is no end in sight when faced with a headwind (except for doing a U-turn I guess).

Twice I was hit by cars. Oh, did I not mention that yet? Fortunately I was not seriously injured. The first encounter broke the index finger on my left hand and the second collision somehow destroyed both of my wheels but didn't harm the frame. The driver's insurance bought me a new set of wheels, and within a week I was back on the road again praying harder than ever as the traffic whizzed by me on the narrow winding roads of Japan.

Biking is probably the most dangerous of the three events as well. I suppose you could drown if something horrific happened and I guess running could lead to tripping and skinning a knee, but cycling beside of cars is downright dangerous. So for that reason, cycling will also improve your relationship with God. You're already going to be sitting there on that bike for six hours at a time. Trucks are going to be screaming past you while the driver is texting, so you might as well use that time to get your affairs in order with your Maker — just in case that driver drops his phone.

Now that I've scared you to death about cycling, I'll tell you that it is also the most peaceful and scenic modes of travel. You'll cover more territory than you ever could while running. You'll certainly see more than just the bottom of a pool, too. It's exhilarating to ride. The fresh air and the wind, the sights, sounds and smells of the city and countryside. Cycling will really put you in touch with nature. You'll notice

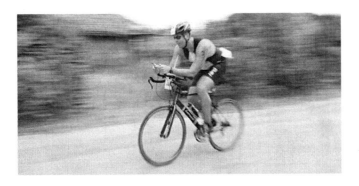

{ *Competing in the Izena 88 triathlon on the Japanese island of Izena in 2008. This 2K swim, 66K bike, 20K run gave me the confidence to go for the full Ironman. It was also the cultural highlight of my three years in Japan.* }

hills that you never noticed driving. You'll smell when it's about to rain, and you'll notice that ... wow, there is a heck of a lot of road kill out there. Biking is also more intense than running. Let me explain. When you run up a hill it is hard, but when you bike up that same hill it is absolutely killer. You have to dig down deep to keep cranking those pedals up a steep hill. Your legs will be screaming and you'll really wish you had just one more gear on your bike. When you run down a hill it is nice, but when you bike down that same hill it's a joyride. Never in swimming or running do you find yourself holding on for dear life as you travel at 40 miles per hour down a hill. Everything is magnified on the bike; the highs are higher and the lows are lower. There's nothing else quite like it.

Cycling the ridiculously long distance that the Ironman requires involves a lot of logistics. Over the course of an 80-100 mile ride you're going to need to plan out a route that allows for water bottle refills. A favorite convenience store or drink machine is the perfect way to stretch for a moment and enjoy a break from the saddle for a minute or two. You'll also probably need a few toilet breaks on a ride that lasts for more than three or four hours (more on that topic later).

{ TIP: DUCT TAPE GOO PACKS TO THE FRAME OF YOUR BIKE. I TAPED 8 GOO PACKS THERE ON RACE DAY. YOU CAN TEAR ONE OFF AND EAT IT WITHOUT HAVING TO DIG THROUGH A BACK POCKET. }

Taking in plenty of calories is extremely important on the bike. Maybe even the most important aspect of an Ironman bike ride. If you're not taking in plenty of nutritious calories while you're biking then you will run flat out of gas during the run. This is often referred to as "bonking." You won't always feel hungry on the bike. In fact, it's rare if you do. But the calories are important for later, so you're going to have to make yourself eat. The best way to do this is to eat a very small portion at regular intervals.

I've heard of a lot of triathletes eating every 15 minutes on the bike. That was a little more than I could do. I found that eating every 30 minutes worked well for me. Every half hour whether I was hungry or not or whether I felt like puking or not, I would eat something. My normal routine was to alternate between a goo pack and a solid. My solids were usually energy bars, peanut butter sandwiches, or bananas.

It's very important to experiment with all sorts of combinations during training. Figure out what you can eat and keep down and what combinations work best for you. Sometimes you'll be surprised to find that some foods that sound great at mile 10 will be a disaster at mile 70, and vice versa.

The important thing is for your body to know that calories are still pouring in at regular intervals. This will keep your body from freaking out and tapping into your body's reserve tanks. If your body thinks that this is some all-out life or death struggle, then it will burn up your energy reserves. When this happens, your recovery time will take days, or even weeks. You might be able to still finish the bike ride without eating, but you will take exceptionally longer to recover, and you certainly won't be in any condition to run a marathon after the ride. But by eating in regular intervals throughout the bike ride you will drastically shorten your recovery time, and you'll even start to actually want to go for a little jog after you put the bike away.

One more point to touch on about nutrition on the bike. Hydration. You cannot do an Ironman on water alone. You're going to need electrolytes. You're going to need sports drinks or salt tablets. Your body is pouring out salts and electrolytes at an alarming rate during a long bike ride in the hot sun. If you're only filling it back up with water you run the risk of getting your body's electrolytes way out of balance.

They make wonderful supplements on the market to aid in this. I used electrolyte tablets regularly. Just drop one or two in a bottle of water and they would dissolve like antacid medicine in about 60 seconds. They come in different flavors and they put the salts that you need back in you. These are handy to carry on a long ride just in case the only hydration source you have is a garden hose or a water fountain somewhere.

The 112-mile leg is a long way to bike, but remember, if you can bike 10 miles this weekend then next weekend you could certainly do 12, and the week after that you could ... you get the idea. Do not get discouraged. The training takes a long time, but you can work your way up to the mileage. Besides, most Ironman venues are booked nine-12 months in advance. So from the time you register and pay to enter an Ironman, you'll have about a year to train. It works out perfect that way. You will have already committed yourself financially (during a moment of temporary insanity), and now all you've got is time. So start training.

{ TIP: GET AEROBARS! THIS REALLY CAN'T BE OVER-EMPHASIZED. THEY TAKE THE STRAIN OFF YOUR SHOULDERS, ARMS, AND HANDS, AND ALLOW YOU TO REST ON YOUR ELBOWS. }

One last word on training for the bike. There will come a time in your training that you just feel like the road is conquering you instead of you conquering it. You'll feel beat down and discouraged. After hammering out 75 miles and being faced with yet another hill, your legs might get a mind of their own and decide to stop pedaling. At times like this (of which I can clearly remember two), I did something completely involuntarily. I talked to myself. Out loud. I never planned on doing this and never would have thought it would have actually helped. But when that moment came and I was hitting the wall I actually said out loud, "Do you want to be an Ironman?"

"Do you want to be an Ironman?"

Now this may seem crazy to you as you sit in a bookstore with a cup of coffee in your hand. Once you've pedaled for hour after hour in the hot sun, dodged traffic, battled dehydration and released your bladder while coasting down hill, however, talking to yourself out loud might just be the least crazy thing you do all day. Hearing a voice ask me that question out loud startled me back into the reality of what I was doing. The magnitude of what I was attempting hit me. Oh yeah, I'm training to do

{ TIP: PORT-A-POTTIES ARE FOR #2; COASTING DOWNHILL IS FOR #1. }

an Ironman! It gave me goose bumps. Suddenly, I came up off the saddle and cranked out a few more miles and a few more hills with a newfound energy.

{BIKING IN JAPAN}

Training for an Ironman is hard enough, but having to train in Okinawa, Japan, offers a whole new set of challenges. Narrow winding roads that careen down the side of jagged mountains are just the beginning. Then there's the fact that many of the roads are single lane. And shoulder? Negative. These interior roads drop off abruptly into dense jungle.

It was a gorgeous sunny day without a cloud in the sky. I was full of energy and ready to put my new bike to the test, so I began riding toward one of the best climbs on the island. Struggling up the steep climb (and being a complete newbie to the world of cycling) I sought relief by shifting gears as I hammered my way up this mountain. With only about 100 yards to go I broke my chain! This was to be the beginning of a very big lesson in cycling.

I was about 25 miles from home and I had no idea how to fix my chain. Flat tires were something I was prepared for, but I had never guessed that I could break a chain. So I coasted down the harrowing mountainside and rolled about a quarter of the way up the next hill before I had to get off and push. I repeated this process about three or four more times. Passing vehicles were few and far between but I tried to thumb a ride from cars that passed and I hoped that my thumb up in the air wasn't some sort of vulgar insult in Japanese. If you've ever seen a picture or clip from an Ironman and someone is pushing

or carrying their bike and they are barefoot, here is the reason —
certain cycling shoes are almost impossible to walk in. They are
designed to clip into the bike's pedals, not be walked around in,
and certainly not to walk for 25 miles back home in.

At the first business I came to (after about five miles
of walking/coasting), I went inside and dazzled the locals with
my mastery of the local language. And by that I mean that I
managed to say, "Konichiwa," and then tried to make arm and
hand gestures to indicate that I needed a taxi because my bike
was broken. 4,000 yen later, I was back home with a few solid
lessons learned:

> 1. Carry a chain tool and a few spare links.
> 2. Carry a cell phone.
> 3. Don't shift gears so hard while pedaling up a hill.
> 4. Cancel all plans to hitchhike across Japan.

The one main road that is flat and well marked and
actually has a shoulder on it is called 58. This road parallels the
coastline on the West side of Okinawa and is a popular road
for every cyclist on the island. I know this for a fact. I saw each
and every one of them as they passed me. The only "cyclists"
that I ever passed in Japan were riding bikes with large baskets
full of groceries on them.

There are however, a few problems with good old
highway 58. First is the fact that every now and again there
will be a telephone pole in the road. Read that last sentence
again. No, it is not a typo. It is all too common to place a

telephone pole in the road in areas where there is no shoulder and no sidewalk. If you enjoy video games like Mario Kart, you'll probably love cycling in Okinawa. After you've dodged the telephone pole you need watch out for the metal grates that run across the entire length of the road. They are there for water drainage and usually they can be found at intersections.

Returning from a 40-mile ride one day, it started raining when I was about two miles from home. The rain gave me a burst of motivation and energy as I crested a hill and passed all the stopped cars at a traffic light. The light turned green just as I got to the front of the line. Perfect! I shifted gears and started to hammer away on my pedals. The light drizzle was beading up on my sunglasses as I prepared to start down hill. I caught notice of the metal grate about 0.2 seconds before it disappeared under my front wheel and both wheels of my bike slid out from under me to the left. Before I could blink, I was laying on my right side and sliding across the middle of the busy intersection, still holding onto my bike. My derailleur was smashed beyond repair, and I was a little scraped up, but I finished my ride home and quickly ran four miles before the adrenaline and shock from the crash wore off.

Part of the problem with cycling in Okinawa is that it is just too beautiful! You're riding beside breathtaking clear blue oceans but you're afraid to even look at them because Grey Hound buses are passing you so close on the other side that you can feel the heat reflecting off their shiny metal surface. You dare not blink or glance at the scenery until you're stopped at a light. Most of the time I was praying and fearing for my life. I had a very close call once in a tunnel that cost me a little bit of skin from my knuckles and shoulder as I was forced to lean in against the side of the tunnel wall. And a couple of times I was bounced off of car hoods — escaping with only minor damage.

During all this, a friend from my church, whom I had done two triathlons alongside of, was hit by a drunk driver one morning and suffered from a broken back and pelvis. She was thrown 40 feet through the air and is lucky to be alive. I discovered the relative safety of the long, empty road that circled the runway at the Air Force base, and I spent many, many hours riding laps around that eight-mile loop. Sure, the scenery wasn't as good, but after all this was my workout; if I wanted scenery I'd go lay on the beach.

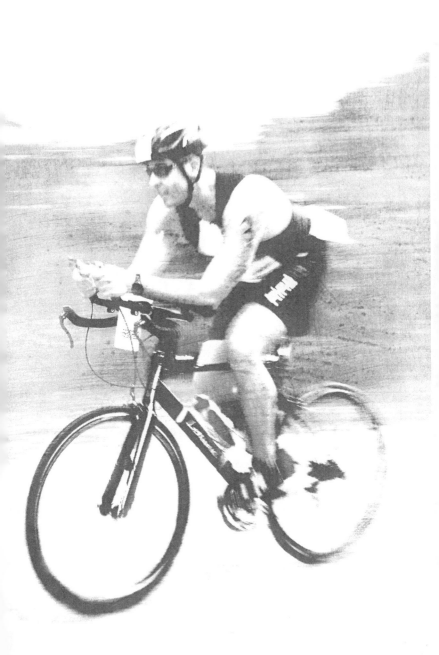

CHAPTER 12

THE RUN

"Don't run with your legs; run with your heart...The human body has limitations; the human spirit is boundless." — Dean Karnazes

I actually felt great through the swim, and I was shocked at how I still felt pretty good coming off the bike. My legs were still strong. My stomach was fine. I was still smiling. My attitude was great; heck, all I had left was just the last of the three events and I would be an Ironman! I came jogging out of T2 (insider jargon for the bike-to-run transition) and I saw my family cheering so I slowed beside of them for a moment. They said things like, "You look great! You can do it, Dave!" And then I heard myself say, "All I've got left to do is run a marathon." I

{ TIP: A SUN VISOR WILL LET HEAT ESCAPE, BUT A CAP CAN HOLD A COLD SPONGE UNDER IT. }

think that when I heard those words the weight of what I was doing settled fully on me. A marathon? Is that all? I'd already been moving for the past nine and a half hours.

It was almost dinnertime. The sun was getting lower in the sky. I felt like getting a shower and relaxing with family and friends. But wait, I still had just this one last thing to do. I

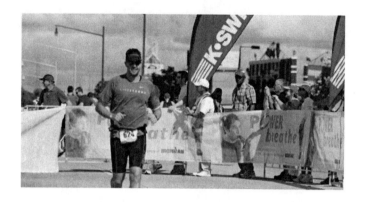

{ *Fresh off the bike with only 26.2 miles between me and that finisher's medal. I was still feeling good – I don't think I realized the long night I had ahead of me.* }

still had to run a stinking marathon!

The run is where an Ironman is made. Since the sport of triathlon is cumulative, the whole of the event is so much greater than the sum of its three parts. It's not just a matter of swimming 2.4 miles, biking 112 miles and running 26.2 miles. It's a matter of doing them all together, back-to-back-to-back. The run is the part of the day in which the swim and bike catch up with you. It's the part of the day when the sun bids you farewell along with most of the fans. The excitement and adrenaline that was there at the swim start that morning is long gone. The wacky signs that spectators were waving along the bike course are nowhere to be seen anymore. The fun and games are over. Now it's just you, out there on your own to finish this thing. Oh, sure, there is an awesome crowd at the finish line with lights, music, police roadblocks and an announcer waiting to call out your name. But that is only the final 0.2 miles. The 26 miles leading up to that will wander through residential areas, country roads and bad sections of town where no one is aware that there are idiots like you on the road trying to run a marathon in the dark.

You'll have several hours out there either by yourself or with a few other runners of a similar pace. You'll use that time to imagine the finish line and what it will be like. You'll use that time to reflect on all that training that you did, and how it's all come down to this and how you're so close to finishing it. You'll be keeping an eye on your watch and doing the mental math that either results in confidence or else a panic that requires you to pick up the pace.

In an Ironman Triathlon it is illegal for headphones to be worn during the race. When I first read that rule it really ticked me off. I love running with my music, making playlists on my iPod or listening to audiobooks or podcasts. I learned so much in all my training. You could earn a degree with all that time you'll spend training.

So I was seriously bummed that I would have to do the whole race without my beloved iPod. But by race day I had begun to respect that rule. And now in hindsight I'm really thankful for it. There is no escapism allowed in an Ironman. You are forced to be in the moment. You can't just listen to music and zone out. If they allowed that then what would be next? Portable DVD players and video games. Pretty soon you'd be able to do the whole thing while watching season four of Scrubs. No music. Period. If you want to be an Ironman you have to do it the old fashioned way.

Who knows, maybe in the absence of music you'll be forced to actually talk to someone else who is running. You might be able to hear complete strangers cheering for you by name (because your race number will also have your first name on it — clever, huh?), and without headphones you might even find yourself encouraging those less fortunate racers who are limping, puking or still headed out on the course when you're on your way back in. This is part of the unmistakable spirit of an Ironman. There's camaraderie and a friendly willingness to help and encourage. No one is out to win at your expense. It is more of an atmosphere of everyone being in this thing together. The only person you're really competing against is yourself.

One nice thing about training for an Ironman is that you don't even have to run as much as someone training only for a marathon. This is because all that swimming and biking you're doing is also increasing your overall fitness. It will help you in your run.

Another reason is that you are not training for a marathon. You're not training for three separate events. It is imperative that you view triathlon as one sport. You are not training for three events: a swim, a bike and a run. You are training for one triathlon. If you tried to train sufficiently for the three individual disciplines all at once you would wreck yourself.

And a final reason that you're weekly mileage is less than a marathon runner's is for recovery and prevention of injury. Training for an Ironman takes a serious toll on your body. You're going to need to schedule plenty of rest and recovery. If you must err, then err on the side of undertraining. It is better to undertrain than to overtrain. If you undertrain the result is that your overall time will be a little slower that you'd like.

{ TIP: PUT DRY SOCKS AND SHOE POWDER IN YOUR RUNNING SPECIAL NEEDS BAG. IF IT RAINED DURING MILE 4, YOU CAN STILL RE-GAIN DRY FEET FOR MILES 14-26. }

But if you overtrain then the result will be an injury that keeps you from finishing altogether.

When I trained for the Lincoln Marathon in 2007, I followed a marathon training plan that I found online. It required me to do two 18-mile runs before I began my taper. But when I trained for the Ironman my longest run was 15 miles.

Most humans don't have the joints to run 26 miles everyday. There comes a point in your training where you start destroying instead of strengthening. Sure, there's a handful of runners out there that have the joints for that, but if you're like most people you're going to have knee pain, shin splints, or stress fractures if you go too far and too hard. I was constantly walking the fine line between not training enough and injuring my knee from running. I had already had three knee surgeries before I discovered the sport of triathlon (thanks to three seasons of soccer per year throughout high school).

For this reason, I knew from the beginning that my strategy would have to be to tread light. Of course, I still had to train and I still had to run. I still went for a two hour run nearly every week. But I didn't grind it into the ground either. If I was going to tear my knee up I was going to do it on race day. I had made peace with the idea of destroying my body on race day in order to get across that finish line. But I didn't want to destroy myself in training and not even make it to the race.

I figured that if I could do all those long months of training, pay the $500 to enter the race, buy the tri bike, buy the airline ticket and travel 6,000 miles and have friends and family travel in order to watch me, then there would be nothing that was going to keep me from finishing. I didn't care if it took me 24 hours to finish. Even if the finish line had packed up and gone home and the next morning's commuters were driving to work, I was going to cross that finish line! I would have crawled across the finish line with two torn up knees and blood coming out of my ears if I had to. That's the kind of passion and determination I had for becoming an Ironman. That is the passion and determination that nearly everyone in the race has. And that is precisely what makes it so easy to overtrain.

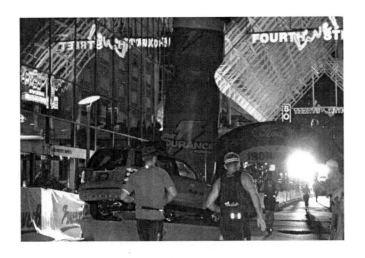

{ *The sweetest sight ever – an Ironman finish line! With only 100 yards to go, a very long day is coming to an end. (Me on the left, Lance on the right.)* }

With that kind of passion and enthusiasm pumping through your veins, it can be torture to force yourself not to run on a perfectly good training day. You might feel great and want nothing more than to lace up your running shoes and strap on your new heart rate monitor. But if you just ran 12 miles the day before or if you plan on biking 80 miles the next day then the best option for you is to find a good book to read or take the kids to the movies. Your joints need rest; they need to recover. Save all that die-hard enthusiasm for race day. You'll be glad you did.

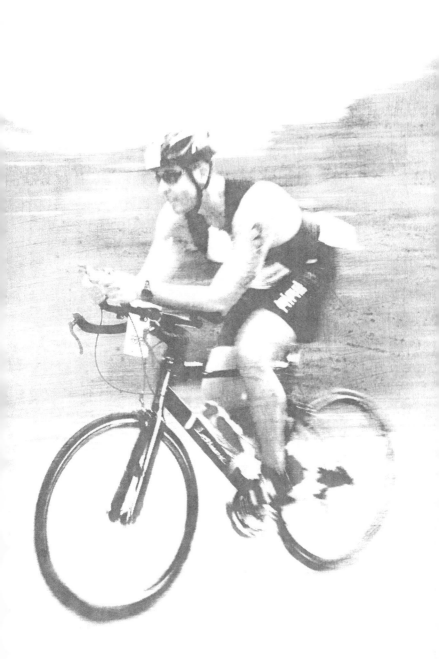

CHAPTER 13

THE SETBACK

"Every noble work is at first impossible." — Thomas Carlyle

The amazing thing about going under for a surgery is that it feels like one second after you close your eyes they are waking you back up again. You're groggy and you can't believe that it's over. You feel like you were given anesthesia only moments ago, but the doctor is standing there looking a little exhausted and he's telling you that everything went great.

I know this routine pretty well. I've gone through this whole thing three times for my right knee. The first two were uneventful. Rest, recovery and rehab, and I was back at it — running and playing soccer again. But the third time I woke up groggy, and the doctor stood there to tell me how it all went, things were a little different. "Well," he started, "we noticed a little something missing while we were looking around in there."

Of course I'm still a little woozy and currently mesmerized by the ice chips someone just handed me.

"You do not have an ACL in your right leg anymore," the doc plainly stated. "It's been torn to bits. There's nothing left of it at all."

"Ok. What does that mean?" I asked.

He went on to explain to me that about 50 percent of the people without an ACL never miss it. They continue as normal. But the other half cannot ever run again without it. My mouth gaped open as I stared at him.

"Get some rest," he said. "We'll just have to wait and see which group you fall into."

Lucky for me, I guess I fell into that first group.

Now with most of my meniscus cartilage removed and no ACL at all, I was back running again. And not just jogging around the block, but actually registering for an Ironman. Sure, it had crossed my mind whether this was really the right thing for me to do — considering my knee and all — but I've always been the kind of person to act first and contemplate later. I'd rather use my body for all the accomplishments and miles that it's worth, than simply grow old in a well-preserved body with low mileage.

Twelve weeks before race day, I was so sick that I could not get out of bed. This was supposed to be the peak of my training. I was scheduled to go for 90-mile bike rides for the next two weekends. This was absolutely no time to get sick! I wasn't sure what God's plan was for me, exactly.

So I was in a pretty foul mood as I drove myself to the Emergency Room on a Sunday afternoon that should have been spent on the bike. It didn't take the doctor long to decide that I had pneumonia. Even though I was afraid deep down that he was going to say that, it still hit me pretty hard when I heard him say it.

By this point, I had been training for almost exactly

one year. I had already put so much into this in money, sweat, hours and ice packs, that I couldn't believe I had pneumonia right here in the home stretch. I had come so far and with just a few more workouts I would start the taper process. Ah, the taper. It had seemed like a mirage for so long. You mean the training plan actually wants me to do *less* this week? I was almost there. And now, this.

Pneumonia is not a small bump in the road. It is a potential show-stopper — an infection inside the lungs, and I don't know if you know this or not, but one thing that swimming, biking and running all three have in common is that they all require a lot of breathing. What if I was sick for a month or more? That would have knocked me out of the race completely. If I had gotten sick six months earlier it would not have been a huge deal, but with only two and a half months to go, I was playing with a much smaller margin of error.

The doc sent me down the hall to radiology to have some chest x-rays taken to determine the extent of the infection. After maneuvering through the various poses for the x-ray, I sat there wearing my lead apron while the technician developed the x-ray film. When he returned to the room, he said we were going to have to take another set of x-rays. I asked why and he asked me if I was triathlete.

This completely shocked me. As I sat there coughing and hacking, feeling dizzy with a fever, I certainly did not feel like a triathlete. Triathletes were people on magazine covers.

Only people with sponsors and shaved legs and $6,000 bikes are called triathletes. And here I sat, a complete mess, sick as a dog and missing crucial workouts. Even healthy, I don't think I could have ever referred to myself as a triathlete. Doctors, lawyers, pilots and firemen all have titles that were conferred upon them. There was a moment in their lives where one day they were not a pilot or doctor and the next day they were. But the title triathlete is much more slippery. Heck, even after finishing an Ironman, I still don't feel comfortable calling myself a triathlete.

He told me that my lungs were too big for the x-ray! He would have to do another set of x-rays to get the other side of my lungs on the film, and that in all his years of taking chest x-rays, the only people he had ever seen whose lungs were too big to fit on a single x-ray were triathletes.

I felt like a rock star being photographed as I stood there for my second round of x-rays. I walked out of that hospital with so much confidence I couldn't believe it. Even though I was still sick and was forced to miss two prime weeks of workouts, I think that having to go to the hospital and have those chest x-rays taken actually bolstered my belief that I could do this race. I never would have gotten this surge in self-confidence had I not gotten sick.

During the next few days of bed rest and prescription drugs, I couldn't help but smile at the thought that I had the lungs of a triathlete. (I still had the love handles of an Average Joe, but at least the lungs were in shape). This trip to the ER confirmed for me that my training had indeed paid off already. I had altered my internal organs, for heaven's sake! I was not the same human being that I had been a year before. My insides had changed and even a doctor could look inside my chest and guess that I was a triathlete! There was tangible, medical proof that I could do this thing, and I wasn't going to let a little pneumonia stand in my way. God had brought me through this setback with more confidence and assurance than I ever had before.

You will, no doubt, encounter similar setbacks in your training. You might get sick or injured. You might get hit by a car, business trips, final exams, or typhoons. The kids will get sick. The in-laws will visit. Your knees will hurt. I had all of those. But if you keep your eyes on the ultimate goal of crossing the finish line then you can get past whatever comes your way.

Ironman is all about endurance and overcoming the odds. This is not just true of the race day. It is true of the entire training experience. Overcoming odds is a crucial part of the Ironman way of thinking, way of racing and ultimately, the Ironman way of living.

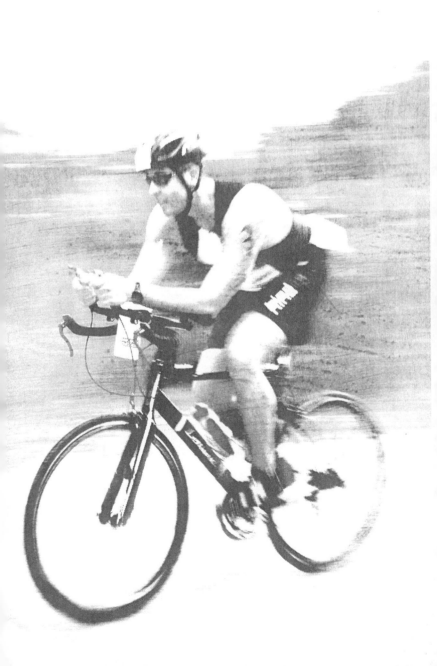

CHAPTER 14

THE AID STATION

"Don't ask how; that will cut your desire off at the knees. How is never the right question; how is a faithless question."

—*John Eldredge*

As you run an Ironman (or even a 10K for that matter), you experience the desire to see an aid station out in front of you. Your eyes scan the horizon on the road ahead of you. Your mouth and throat are dry and you're beginning to doubt if there's even an aid station out there. You want badly to see one, to run towards it and to have it quench your thirst and equip you to carry on.

Authors like Donald Miller see God as the Writer. Artists view God as the Master Painter. To a builder God is the Great Architect, and others have viewed God as the Designer, Shepherd, Defender, or Fisherman. To me, God became my Aid Station.

I discovered that God is very much like these aid stations. He prepares a table before me. My cup runs over. He restores my soul. The thing about these aid stations is that they are not always located right where you want them to be. Sometimes you've been pedaling for miles with empty water bottles, and you're questioning their very existence. At other times things are going well, you feel great, and you fly right by one without even stopping. You think, "Who needs one now? I'm just fine on my own."

Ironman taught me a lot about trust and faith over the course of the one year I spent training for it and then the day I spent racing it. I was full of doubt along the way. Would there be a debilitating injury? Would I get sick? Would I be able to finish at all? Would I crash? But it was trust (or at least hope) that kept me going, kept me moving towards the finish line.

I think there's a certain amount of trust that goes into just registering for an Ironman. You have to have some faith that you're not just throwing away your $500 registration fee. You have to believe that you might actually be able to pull this thing off.

Trust is not necessarily something that happens all at once. Like becoming an Ironman, trusting in God is something you do a little bit more of every day. Becoming an Ironman, much like trusting in God, is a process that we get better at with practice. I had to learn to trust in God just the same way I had to trust in the aid stations. God would be there to provide for me. But I had to learn to trust in His timing and in His location. I grew closer to God through my training. There were hundreds upon hundreds of beautiful miles of His creation that I enjoyed as I biked. God's scenery was breathtaking. The mountains, trees, birds and sunrises brought me closer to my Creator. (And the speeding cars brought me inches closer to actually meeting Him!) Somewhere along the course of my training I started talking to God. Out loud. At first this felt strange, but then it became a part of my routine. And why not? I'm out here on the road, either biking or jogging for hours and hours with no one else around. It was awesome.

Workouts became a quiet time when it would just be God and I. Then my friend Drew suggested that I try listening to an Andy Stanley podcast one time. This revolutionized both my training runs and my spiritual life! I could listen to two podcasts per run and I'd lose track of time, hanging on each word of his message, I'd be laughing or smiling, or nodding in agreement as I ran (not caring how you look is a prerequisite for triathlons).

Then I'd get home and share what I'd heard with Kerry, and talk about how I felt my life was changing. Something weird was going on with me. I think I was starting to ... what do people call it? Oh yeah, "get closer to God." And it was actually cool.

Ironman is a metaphor for the journey of life and the ups and downs and pains and joys along the way, and God was like the aid stations that gave me strength and nourishment along the way. My life was starting to come together. Both physically and spiritually, things were improving.

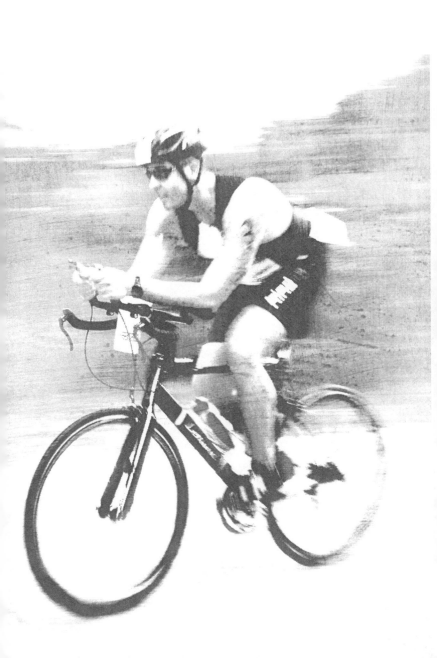

CHAPTER 15

THE TAPER

"Success is to be measured not so much by the position that one has reached in life as by the obstacles which he has overcome."
— *Booker T. Washington*

Tapering off your mileage as you get close to race day is imperative to Ironman training. It requires a mentality of pulling back on the reigns and not letting your body go all out during those last weeks of training. This is going to be harder than it sounds. After months of pushing your limits, it won't be easy to make yourself rest.

My Ironman taper was eight weeks long. That doesn't mean that I did nothing for eight weeks. Far from it. I still did some pretty long workouts during that time, but each was gradually becoming shorter and shorter.

For over a year I had been stretching and pushing myself to go farther, farther, farther. Swim just five more laps, bike just 10 more miles, run just 30 more minutes. That was my life for months and months. Then when I hit the day on the calendar when my Ironman was only eight weeks away everything changed. Now I had to think differently. Now I had to actually stop myself instead of pushing myself. Do five less laps, stop 15 miles short, run 30 minutes less.

An eerie feeling sets in that you're doing it all wrong, that you're cheating or something. You start to feel guilty for not pushing yourself to the verge of heatstroke. And then you have a really bizarre feeling — energy. For the past six months I had been chronically fatigued. My body had forgotten what it's like to not be utterly exhausted. But now as I started to taper, my energy level gradually began to return.

Four weeks into an eight-week taper you start to feel really good. In fact you are dying to run. I found myself wishing that the Ironman were the very next day. Your body is healing itself. Joints are recovering. Energy is back. The plan comes together perfectly. By the week before the Ironman you will be chomping at the bit. Odds are that you will have never been in that level of fitness before in your life. You'll feel invincible, like you could run right through a wall. Save it. You're going to need that level of energy and enthusiasm 80 miles into the bike ride when you realize you still have to ride for 32 more miles just to get to the starting line of a marathon.

For me, it wasn't until this taper period that I really started to feel optimistic about finishing. When the Ironman was just two weeks away I was feeling at my peak. For over a year, I had been saying to myself, "I wonder if I can do this." Now I was actually starting to say, "You know, I think that I can do this."

During these final two weeks as you prepare to travel to your race, you will begin to look at everything a whole new way. Anyone who sneezes or coughs around you is your sworn enemy, and if they don't cover their mouth you will not hesitate to switch tables, restaurants, or movie theaters. You become hyper aware of anything that could derail your Ironman goal.

Also, during these last few weeks, you'll want to taper your calorie intake as well. You might have done fine eating three helpings of pasta before your 90-mile bike ride, but now that you're only biking 25 miles you might want to ease off of the carbs as well as the miles.

The notable exception to this however, is the night before the race. This is the perfect, one and only time, when you might seriously want to consider eating everything that sounds good to you. The night before my Ironman I went out to a local restaurant with about 15 close friends and family members. I ordered the chicken and fettuccini Alfredo, as well as a gourmet cheeseburger, and don't forget the cheese fries and — of course — salad and bread. I felt like I wanted all the calories there when I woke up in the morning, because I knew there wouldn't be much going in the entire next day.

{ TRAINING LOG }

Now that I've covered the swim, bike and run, along
with the setback and the taper, I want to show you the exact
amount of training that I did.

To show other Average Joes like me exactly how they
too can complete an Ironman is the entire reason I wrote this
book. As you look at my training chart below you'll notice that
it really isn't that time consuming. Whereas other books call for
five to six workouts and average 20 or more hours of training
per week, you'll see that I typically did three to four workouts at
roughly eight to 12 hours per week.

My plan below allows for working a full-time job
with long hours, taking night classes and still spending
quality time with family.

PLEASE KEEP TWO THINGS IN MIND AS YOU LOOK AT THIS CHART:

*I am not a professional coach; this is simply the plan that I followed
and made up as I went. But hey, it worked for me! It got me across
the finish line. And if you're not trying to win the race then this is the
plan you're looking for. It is designed for Average Joes who are looking
to get that finisher's medal.*

*I did not start from scratch at week 24. I had been training for a half
iron-distance race for several months, completed that tri and then rolled
into this training for the full distance. So if you've been doing nothing
but watching TV for a year, please don't think you can start cold on
week 24.*

141

* Indicates the longest workout of your life. The taper begins after this.

Weeks Out	Mon	Tues	Wed	Thur	Fri	Sat	Sun
24	5 mile run		swim 30 laps	3 mile run		25 mile bike	
23		swim 30 laps	swim 30 laps				30 mile bike
22	swim 40 laps		1 hr bike/30 min run			40 mile bike	
21	6 mile run		1 hr bike			10 mile run	
20			1 hr bike/30 min run		swim 30 laps	50 mile bike	
19			6 mile run	swim 40 laps		50 mile bike/30 min run	
18	swim 50 laps	3 mile run		2 hr bike/30 min run		60 mile bike	80 mile bike
17	4 mile run		swim 40 laps	2 hr bike/30 min run			12 mile run
16			swim 40 laps	3 hr bike/30 min run	5 mile run		
15	swim 50 laps		1 hr bike/30 min run				75 mile bike
14		5 mile run	swim 60 laps			65 mile bike/30 min run	
13	12 mile run		swim 60 laps	1 hr bike/30 min run			80 mile bike
12	Sick	Sick	Sick	Sick	Sick		Sick
11	Sick	Sick	Sick	Sick	4 mile run		70 mile bike
10		5 mile run	swim 60 laps	swim 60 laps	7 mile run		80 mile bike
9			3 hr bike/30 min run	swim 80 laps	15 mile run		
8	3 mile run		swim 60 laps	1 hr bike/30 min run		96 mile bike*	
7		5 mile run		swim 50 laps		1 hr bike/30 min run	75 mile bike
6		6 mile run		swim 40 laps		65 mile bike/30 min run	
5	5 mile run		swim 40 laps	1 hr bike/30 min run		60 mile bike	
4	4 mile run		swim 40 laps			40 mile bike	6 mile run
3			swim 30 laps	1 hr bike/30 min run		30 mile bike	4 mile run
2		8 mile run		swim 30 laps		30 mile bike/3 mile run	4 mile run
1	3 mile run		swim 20 laps			20 mile bike	

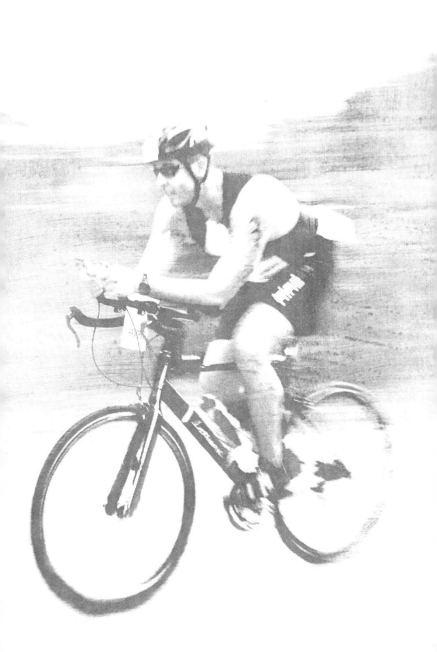

CHAPTER 16

THE TRANSITION

"All you need is ignorance and confidence and the success is sure."
— Mark Twain

Transition is sometimes referred to as the fourth event of a triathlon. There is even a market for transition gear. They sell special mats to stand on, and special laces you don't have to tie. There are volunteers who will help you out of your wetsuit once you finish the swim. There are even volunteers standing ready with their hands covered in sunscreen. They will slap it on your shoulders and neck as you run by them. You'll even see pros and top age-groupers take their feet out of their shoes while they are still on the bike because they can run faster barefoot than they can in their cycling shoes.

{ **TIP: AN UNWRAPPED GRANOLA BAR WILL STICK NICELY TO YOUR HANDLEBARS. THIS MAKES IT QUICK AND EASY TO EAT DURING YOUR RIDE.** }

In the second sprint triathlon that I did I decided to make my transitions as fast as possible. So I bought speed laces for my shoes and decided to forgo socks. Who has time to wrestle a sock on over a wet and dirty foot anyway? When I crossed that finish line there were bloodstains seeping through the heels of my shoes. I guess that extra minute it takes to put on socks would have been a good investment after all.

My advice for your transitions is to take them slow. Don't be in a hurry. Forgetting a simple item like socks or sunscreen might prove to be a costly mistake a few hours down the road.

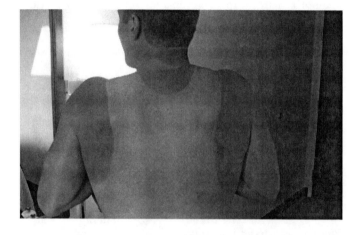

{ *My buddy Lance demonstrates why you should take the time to put on sunscreen during transition. This picture was taken the day after the Ironman.* }

I've heard stories of people getting massages during their transitions. Now, this might be taking it a bit too far, but I'm sure these folks didn't forget anything either. I wasn't quite that nonchalant with my transitions but I like the idea (in theory).

Sometimes you might see a bright colored helium balloon tied to a bicycle at T1 (insider jargon for the swim-to-bike transition). This is to help this person quickly find their bike amidst the sea of cycles. When I first saw this, I thought that it was a pretty clever idea. After all, there are about 3,000 bikes and instead of hunting for your row and number you could just run right to the balloon. This might shave a good five to 10 seconds off your time (probably the same five to 10 seconds it takes to untie the balloon from your bike).

I chose a different strategy to make finding my bike easier; I waited until about 75 percent of the bikes were gone before I exited the water. You would not believe how easy it was to find my bike. So don't tie a balloon to your bike unless you know you're a fast swimmer. You

{ **TIP: TRY TO REMEMBER NOT TO BLOW YOUR NOSE AS YOU GET OUT OF THE WATER - YOUR PICTURE IS BEING TAKEN.** }

don't want a balloon on your bike if it's the only bike left.

If your swim exit takes you across sand it might be a good idea to have a jug of fresh water in your transition gear. I did this when I raced the Izena 88 in Japan and it definitely came in handy. I poured the water over my feet before putting on my socks and cycling shoes. Free from sand and saltwater, my feet felt great the entire day.

Also, along with your running shoes you can leave an insulated lunch box with an ice-cold drink of your choice in it. Pick something other than sports drink or water since this will be available at every aid station along the way. It can be a real boost to your morale after having biked 112 miles to have a half-frozen soda waiting for you.

Finally, those two minutes in which you sit down and lace up your shoes during transition are likely to be the only time in the whole day that you aren't kicking, pedaling, or running. This might be a good time to relieve your bladder of some of the excess weight it's been carrying around. I know, this sounds gross, but I'm just saying, those port-a-potty lines are long, and that tri suit is hard to get on and off. Just saying.

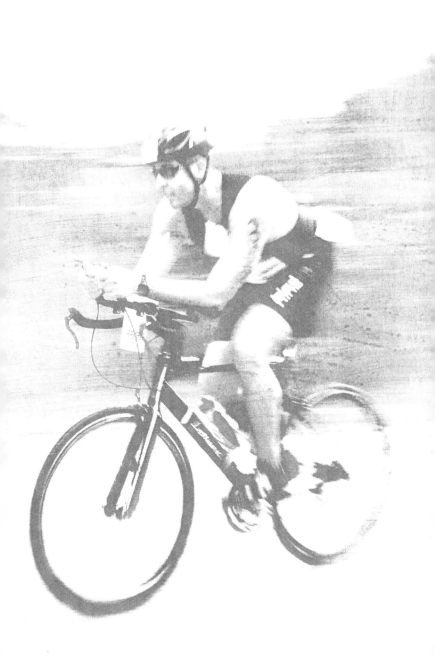

CHAPTER 17

THE TRAVEL

"Life is either a daring adventure or it is nothing." — Helen Keller

By now you've finished your training and your tapering. You've booked your hotel room, planned out some meals and called a friend or two in the area. You're ready to make The Trip.

The logistics that go into traveling to an Ironman Triathlon can be just about as daunting as the race itself. It is in this one area (and only this one) that I believe I can speak with a fair amount of expertise. For few people have traveled farther to race in an Ironman than I did when I flew from the tiny island of Okinawa, Japan, to Louisville, Kentucky.

For three days I had attempted to fly stand-by and hop on an open seat in an Air Force cargo plane. We call this flying Space Available, and for me there was zero space available. I packed my bags, took apart my bike and packed it neatly into a travel case, kissed my wife and kids goodbye, and drove myself to the passenger terminal to anxiously wait and see if I could hop in the back of a cargo plane.

A few hours later I lugged all my bags and bike back home. Having just said goodbye to the family, this really did screw with the kids. Especially when I went through this charade three days in a row.

Finally, I came to terms with the $1,500 airline ticket I would have to buy. I kissed my wife and kids goodbye for a fourth time as they dropped me off at the airport.

If you happen to be flying to your race, I cannot emphasize enough how perfect of an opportunity that flight will be to cash in on however many frequent flyer rewards, bonus points, tokens, coupons and miles you have stored up. Because if you ever fly first class in your life, make it on the flight to your Ironman.

{ TIP: DEFLATE YOUR BIKE TIRES WHEN TRAVELING ON AN AIRPLANE. THE DEPRESSURIZED BAGGAGE COMPARTMENT COULD CAUSE AN INFLATED TUBE TO RUPTURE. }

I say this for several reasons. The primary reason I upgraded to first class on my flight from Tokyo to Atlanta was in order to get as far away as possible from the coughing, sneezing, runny noses that were plotting to crawl all over me, in an attempt to sabotage my plans for a healthy race day.

I reasoned that with more space between myself and the other passengers, I would be less likely to catch those germs that notoriously attack us on airplanes. For this reason I also drank a vitamin C drink (about every four hours or so) that claims to boost your immune system.

Disclaimer: Ordinarily, I am not this much of a

germaphobe. But after putting in that amount of time, effort and money, I became hyper-aware of anything that had the potential to derail my plans.

And, just in case you're not already thoroughly convinced, you will also get more rest in a first class seat. This sleep can help boost your immune system and combat the effects of jet lag. Plus, you're going to eat way better and be more relaxed and focused on your race.

Unlike packing for a business trip or family vacation, traveling to the destination of your Ironman requires that you bring your bike. There are numerous businesses springing up to help triathletes ship their bikes from their homes to the races. Whether you use one of these services or you take it yourself like I did, I definitely recommend taking it by a bike shop for a pre-race tune up once you arrive at your destination.

The importance of having your bike professionally fit to your body cannot be overstated. By taking your bike to a bike shop and having a professional make minute adjustments, you will be shocked at how much more comfortable and efficient you become at cycling. Even a saddle that is moved one millimeter forward can make a huge difference. Your back and neck will be glad you took the time to have this done when you've been riding for six hours. And be sure to mark these positions on your bike with a permanent marker so that you can put it back together precisely the same way after taking it apart.

But don't overlook the importance of a last minute tune up by a pro once you get to the city of your race. After flying and getting handled by the velvet gloves of airline baggage handlers, something on your bike might have gotten shook loose and it might need a minor tweak or adjustment. Better safe than sorry. Plus, you'll need to stop by a bike shop anyway to pick up the last minute things you forgot to pack or the CO_2 cartridges that were illegal to take on an airplane. Yep, they make a tire pump that inflates your tube quicker than you can say, Dang, I've got a flat tire! It uses a CO_2 cartridge and it can save you lots of time.

Once you've arrived and had your bike assembled and tuned, you'll want to go for a nice 20-mile (or so) ride. It will probably have been a couple of days since you were able to workout, and going for a short bike ride around the city of your race will help prepare you mentally for the new streets and new climate.

I also highly recommend that you give your pass card to a friend or family member so that they can gain access to the racer's only area. That way they can retrieve your bike for you while you're still running. Going to get your bike is the last thing you'll want to think about after crossing the finish line.

I was also able to get in a very short swim the day prior to the race. This can be of great benefit in that it eliminates another unknown come race day. Get in a practice swim the day prior and you won't be wondering what the temperature of the water is when you're standing at the starting line the next morning. The swim seems to be the part of the triathlon that people fear the most. For some it's the crowd of other swimmers, for some it's the waves or the saltwater. For me it was the current of the river.

River swims are becoming more and more common as Ironman spreads to new venues. They always start by swimming up river — against the current. Then you circle a buoy and swim back to a point farther downstream than you began. This way it sort of all evens out (effort wise).

My fear was that I would jump in the water and swim for 20 minutes and then notice that I had moved backwards five feet. What if I can't swim harder than the current? So the day prior to the race I jumped in the Ohio River to get a feel for how hard I would have to swim in order to move against the current. Much to my surprise, the current was not that bad. I stayed close to the shoreline and made decent progress. That five-minute swim the day prior to the race was a huge confidence booster. I entered the water with confidence on race day, and I highly recommend that everyone take advantage of the Ironman practice swim the day prior to your race.

One last travel tip: if you will be renting a car at your destination, make sure to either bring a bike rack with you or rent a large enough car to accommodate your bike. You're going to be lugging a lot of gear, not to mention family and friends around in that subcompact car rental. Some car rental agencies might even have bike racks for rent.

Lucky for me, the rental company was all out of the compact cars that I had reserved and they were forced to give me a 15-passenger van for the same price. We were now able to put our bikes in the van along with three rows of friends and family.

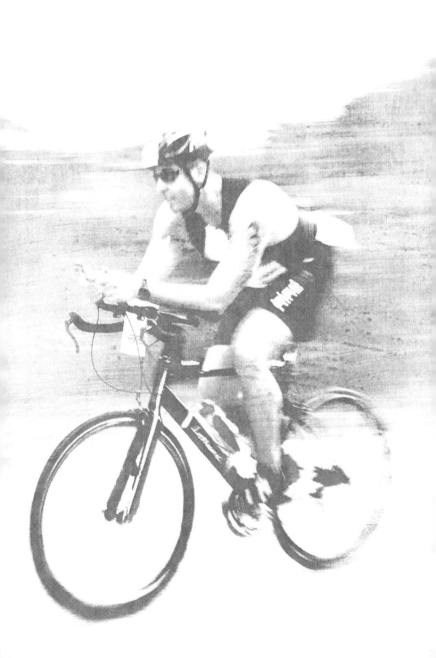

CHAPTER 18

THE RACE

"I wanted to live deep and suck out all the marrow of life"
— Henry David Thoreau

From the moment you arrive in the city where your race is to be held, you're going to feel a definite buzz in the air. You'll be treated like a professional athlete from the time you pick up your race packet until the finisher's medal is hung around your neck.

For me it started when I stood in line to pick up my race number and packet. The very first thing they did was weigh me and test my body fat and hydration. Then they wrote it all down and handed me a card. The lady

{ TIP: ONE PIECE TRI SUITS TAKE LONGER TO REMOVE IF NATURE CALLS. A PINK TRI SUIT IS A RECIPE FOR DISASTER. }

smiled and stated, "13 percent body fat, 54 percent hydrated — you've got no excuses." I knew that anything higher than 50 percent hydration was very good. I'd been chugging water all week to get myself "super hydrated." And well, the 13 percent body fat thrilled me. I had no idea what to expect. I weighed 207 when I started training the year prior. Now I checked in at the race weighing 194. I was excited! That was 13 pounds that

I would not have to lug around with me all day.

The expo can be fun, exciting, and also intimidating. Professional triathletes from all around the world are there with television cameras pointed at them. Bikes are on display that cost more than my car, and there is a heavy sense of anticipation in the air. Everyone can feel the race looming over them. It's a foreboding feeling, but it's one you signed up for. I

{ TIP: COVER YOURSELF IN SUNSCREEN BEFORE PUTTING ON YOUR TRI SUIT. INEVITABLY, THE SUIT WILL MOVE AND SHIFT AND THE NEWLY EXPOSED SKIN WILL BURN. }

walked around the expo looking at all the merchandise with the Ironman logo on it and all the shirts that said "Finisher." I could not bring myself to buy any of them. As badly as I wanted one, I knew that I was not yet an Ironman finisher. I'm not a superstitious person, but I wasn't going to wear anything until I had earned it. Just in case.

That night, my parents and sisters arrived. They flew in from Atlanta or drove over from Virginia. My friend Drew drove up from North Carolina to Kentucky. There was so much anticipation in the air you could taste it. I had never felt better in my entire life. I knew that this was my peak, my prime. I recognized the fact quietly to myself that I would most likely never be in better shape than at this very moment.

I felt like I could run through a brick wall. My taper had paid off big time. I was bursting with energy and couldn't wait to unleash myself that next morning.

We all went out for dinner that night talking and catching up on each other's lives. It had been a long time since we were all together like this. With all of us grown with families of our own and me living in Okinawa, Japan, this Ironman had inadvertently brought the entire family back together again. I felt like the stars were aligned. Like nothing could go wrong. I had come so far and now it was all coming together. We sat around laughing and talking while I ate fettuccini Alfredo and a cheeseburger. I wasn't the least bit concerned with whether or not those calories would get burned off or not.

That night in my hotel room I went through everything in my head one last time, and prayed for God to help me finish what I had already started. Sleep did not come quickly and it did not last long.

Your alarm clock goes off at 3:30 a.m., and it's THE DAY. You've been training and thinking and dreaming about this day for a year now, and today is go-time! For me, the most important aspect of that morning was to have my coffee, some breakfast and my proper morning "movement." I didn't want to be one of those poor souls standing in the long line at the port-a-potty when the announcer declares, "Two minutes until race start." Fortunately, a bagel, banana and some hotel coffee helped me ease into the day.

You drop off your bike and all your gear for biking and running the day prior to the race. The staff support at an Ironman is phenomenal. They treat everyone like a professional athlete. So on the morning of the race, you no longer have to worry about your helmet or your running shoes. It's all been done already.

You take a quick shower to wake up and then put on your tri suit. I recommend waking up early so that you're not rushed. I enjoyed a second cup of coffee, lots of stretching and talking with family and friends as we finished getting ready and drove down to the race start. Once we got down there, we went into the bike area and I inflated my bike tires once more just to top them off. In Louisville, the swim start is about 1.5 miles away from the swim exit/bike start, so along with a couple thousand other nervous and half-asleep people, we started walking down the path. It was still very dark outside at 5:30 a.m., and the line was already a mile long for the swim start and every port-a-potty was surrounded by people waiting to use them. Maybe it was just nerves or maybe it was the gallon of water I had been sipping on in order to hydrate myself — but for whatever reason, I had to go to the bathroom about 10 times before the start of the race. Fortunately for me, there were wooded areas all along the way, and well ... I'm a guy.

Gradually, the sky began to lighten and the announcer began to speak. The National Anthem played.

"Here we go," I thought. "This is it. It's starting. I'm actually about to attempt an Ironman! What have I done?"

The cannon roared and once again I heard U2's Beautiful Day blast out over the speakers as the line I was in began to move.

Swim goggles — on.

Swim cap — on.

Flip–flops — off.

Stopwatch — start.

I leaped off the dock (I thought the best way to start my day would be with a cannonball). I sank down deep into the Ohio River and thought, "Oh no, what if somebody else jumps in on me!" Finally I surfaced and began to swim. I immediately settled into my comfortable, slow, free-style stroke that had become so familiar from all those lunch breaks spent in the pool. Only this time someone had removed all the lane dividers. I was relieved to notice that I was making forward progress against the current. For months I had worried that the current of the river might just hold me in one place no matter how hard I swam.

For me the swim was relaxing. Sure there were moments of getting clawed and kicked, but for the most part I was able to settle into a group of swimmers and just enjoy watching the sun come up over the bank of the river, I saw the Louisville skyline whenever I turned my head to the left for a breath, and swimming underneath all those bridges was enough to keep me distracted. It definitely wasn't boring like staring at the bottom of a pool.

As I exited the water, I was completely off balance and my equilibrium was out of whack. After swimming that distance, there is very little blood in your legs or feet — it's all gone to your arms, so everyone is a little wobbly coming out of the water. Despite having water in my ears, I could hear my name being called out in the crowd. I paused just long enough to see my dad there cheering, and then I saw my mom and sisters. I checked my watch to see that I had completed the swim in 1 hour 39 minutes. I was pumped. I would

{ TIP: THE BEST WAY TO EAT A BANANA WHILE RIDING A BIKE IS TO TAKE A BANANA HALF AND SQUEEZE IT FROM THE BOTTOM UP. }

have been happy to do it in anything under 2 hours. By now the sun was up and it was the beginning of a bright beautiful day. I ran to the tent where I grabbed my bag and found a vacant folding chair.

Transitions are where you really feel like a triathlete. It's always a mentality of never mind what you just did, the only thing that matters now is what you're going to do next. Who cares that you just swam 2.4 miles? No one has a second to waste discussing ancient history like that. Your priority now is simply getting on your socks, cycling shoes, sunglasses and helmet. With the Ohio River still dripping off of me, I grabbed my bike off the rack and started rolling it toward the bike start. Just then, I heard my buddy Lance.

The thing about Lance is that he could sit on a couch eating ice cream for 12 straight months and then go run a marathon. He once spent a summer riding a bicycle from California to Washington, D.C. We met in college where we shared an apartment together, and while I was out running, Lance was busy pledging a fraternity, and even then I couldn't keep up with him when we'd go for a run.

So I never expected to see Lance once the race began. I figured that by the time I stumbled back to the hotel after the race he would have already showered, eaten dinner and been ready to talk me into going out on the town. So when I heard his voice, I was pleasantly surprised. He was just strapping on his helmet and getting his bike off the rack, too. We yelled out a few words to each other about how the swim went pretty well and then I took off on my bike — knowing that he was only about 10 yards behind me and expecting him to pull up beside me at any moment.

It's an exhilarating moment when you take off on the bike in an Ironman triathlon. Intersections are blocked by police cars. Spectators line the sidewalks. Horns, bells, cameras, the works. You ride through the city and see the cars gridlocked and local television stations all around and think, "This is for me. I'm doing something worth stopping traffic over!"

And then I headed out of town.

The crowds gradually get replaced by rolling hills. The sun positions itself directly overhead and before you know it, the pack is gone and it's just you and a few other cyclists trying to crank out those miles and muscle up those hills. This is probably the first moment since waking up that I had to actually take a deep breath, look around and just think. There's plenty of time for that out there on the bike course.

The loop takes you back through town and you can once again hear the bells and horns and clappers getting louder and louder. It wakes you up out of your daydream and you remember where you are and what it's all about. At the 56-mile halfway point you get handed a special needs bag that you packed for yourself the day prior. I had been religiously eating every 30 minutes throughout the entire bike ride, alternating between a goo pack and a bar. So I wasn't exactly hungry as I pilfered through my bag to see if anything I had packed sounded good to eat. My stomach saw only one thing in the bag that it wanted — a Hostess brand little cherry pie. Jackpot! I scarfed that thing down like a man who hadn't eaten in months. It was the most delicious thing I had ever tasted in my life! I tossed the rest of the bag and got back on my bike. I felt renewed, recharged.

Just a few miles later I saw all my family and friends waving and cheering, and my spirits soared. I was rapidly approaching mile 70, but thanks to family, friends and Hostess,

I felt like I was on mile one.

And then I headed out of town.

This time nature cranked up the thermostat. I was covered with white salt from the residue left after my sweat had evaporated. I looked like some kid had dusted the erasers on my black tri suit. I was sucking down the Gatorade and water and just plugging along as best I could.

There were only two times during the entire ride that I actually got off my bike. The first was at mile 56 for the cherry pie in my special needs bag, and the second time was around the 80- or 90-mile mark. My back was aching and my neck was screaming and I just needed to straighten up for a second. So when I spotted a good aid station I pulled over and got off my bike for a moment. I stretched my back and legs, took an ibuprofen and traded in my empty bottles for full ones.

As I started to get back on my bike I saw Lance go zipping by. I had not seen him since we were at the transition tent and I was surprised we were so evenly paced on the bike. I struggled but eventually caught up with him and we talked about the bike course and about the run we had ahead of us. We rode the last 15 or so miles together on the bike, and entered the transition area once again.

I had done the math in my head more than 100 times, always rounding up just to be conservative. Two hours to swim, Eight hours to bike, that still left seven hours to complete the marathon before the midnight cutoff. My goal was always simple – just finish. But now I had finished the swim in less than two hours and biked in fewer than eight, so I knew that the finish line was within reach. I could take my time and enjoy a nice slow jog around Louisville.

My mental plan from the get-go was to view the entire run as simply 26 one-mile runs. It helped tremendously to break it down like that. I mean, who can't do a one mile run? You can always do a one-mile run, right? How about another? And maybe just one more? I was going to go for a one-mile jog, drink some water and repeat — 26.2 times. This plan worked like a charm. I focused on the next aid station. I would just run to the next aid station. I followed the

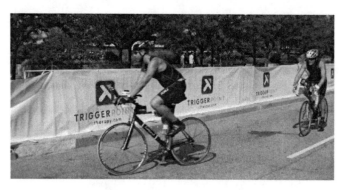

{ *Lance (on the right) and I pulling into T2 after a nice little 112 mile stroll around Kentucky. I was so tired of sitting on that bike that I seriously considered throwing it into the Ohio River.* }

advice that I once heard a pro give, "Never pass an aid station without taking something from it." I put at least some kind of energy in my body at every single aid station. Even if all I could stomach was just one single grape.

Upon arriving at an aid station, I would grab a cup of water or sports drink and a piece of fruit or pretzel and I would walk for about 10 yards while I consumed it. There was no point in splashing and spilling it all over myself by trying to eat and drink on the run. That saves about as much time in the big scheme of things as shaving your legs. If you're not competing for first place, what's the point of shedding a couple more seconds? I enjoyed my pretzel or my grape and allowed myself to walk a few steps at each aid station. Then I'd mentally say to myself, "Ok, let's run one more mile to the next aid station."

{ TIP: PUT IBUPROFEN IN A ZIPLOC BAG AND TAKE IT WITH YOU FOR THE RUN. INEVITABLY, THINGS WILL ACHE, CRAMP, AND SWELL THAT NEVER DID BEFORE. }

The only time during the course of the Ironman that I actually felt discouraged was at the turnaround part of the run. There comes a point on the run course, just a little over the halfway mark, that you find yourself running right through downtown and directly toward the finish line. With only a few yards between myself and the finish line there was a sign for everyone on their "first lap" to make a right turn. There were people running all around me, many were on their second lap. The crowd is going wild, the

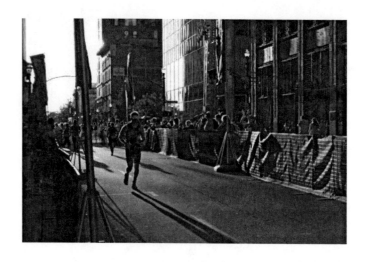

{ *Shadows were growing long as Lance approached the mid-run turn around point. It was crushing to be so near the finish line and have to turn around for another 13 mile run.* }

announcer is calling out the finishers and the music is playing. You glimpse the glory of the Ironman finish line for just a moment and then you must turn right, away from the crowds and the finish line, and do that run all over again.

As soon as you make that right turn you are back out on a random road where you feel isolated and alone. The sun is setting and you know you have a lot of road out there in front of you and that it's going to be a very long night. Being right there at the finish line and turning away to make a second lap is an emotionally daunting moment. It's like glimpsing the Pearly Gates and turning around to make one more trip back through hell.

For me, my entire family was at this halfway point. They tried to cheer and encourage me as they had throughout the entire day. They had been there at the swim before the sun had even come up. They were there for me on the bike loop, and back there for me again in town when I finished the bike and started the run. Now they were there at the turnaround point of the run. I knew I would not see them again until I was back to cross that finish line.

At every step of the way I had worn a smile and joked with friends and family as they cheered me on. I'm the kind of person who thrives under pressure and my optimism and positive attitude usually increase as things get harder. But somewhere along the course of the day my smile must have faded. Sure, I tried to fake it when I saw my family and friends cheering me on at the turn around point; I nodded and smiled and reassured them that I was doing fine. But you can't fool family. They must have seen the discouragement and exhaustion in my eyes when I made that right hand turn.

About one block after that turn around, I heard my name being called. It was easy to hear because there were no crowds or spectators on the empty street I was now running on. I turned around to see my sisters running after me to cheer me on. The tears in their eyes as they looked at me stopped me dead in my tracks. Literally. They said, "David, you WILL do this. You WILL make it. Don't get discouraged. You've come so far and you are ALMOST THERE!" I didn't even know what to say. I was choked up. But their motivation poured over me. I was renewed.

As if the inspirational soundtrack to my life kicked in, I turned and began to run. Not like a man who is tired and beaten, but like a man who knows he's going to achieve his goal. I felt the greatness of my looming achievement and I felt the tears and cheers of everyone that I hold dear drawing me on toward that finish line.

I've often heard my dad say that what kind of man we are is determined by what it takes to make us quit. How much can we take before we decide to give up? That's the question that reveals what we're made of. There's no value in a trophy that is easily won. It's only when we encounter problems and refuse to give up that our victory becomes sweet.

So how much would it take to make me quit? I decided right then to make my answer be, "just a little more." I could always handle just a little bit more.

With a new focus I continued to run. Then somewhere around mile 17 I felt a rumble in my stomach and for the first and only time during the course of the race, I went into a port-a-potty. The process of removing a tri suit from within the confines of a port-a-potty proved to be as daunting as the marathon itself. When I finally wrestled myself free of the spandex prison, my stomach pains had disappeared. The only thing harder than trying to free oneself from a wet triathlon suit is trying to get back into one.

Back on the road again the distance between aid stations seemed to be magically increasing. My legs wanted so badly to stop running but my brain was forcing them to just keep moving forward.

In the absence of music and all my carefully crafted iPod playlists, and without the awesome distractions from cheering fans, I ran in reflective silence. A poem that I had memorized many years prior came flashing back to the forefront of my mind - IF by Rudyard Kipling.

I clung to one particular phrase about holding on, it became my rallying cry: "If you can force your heart and nerve and sinew to serve your turn long after they are gone, and so hold on when there is nothing in you except the will which says to them, 'Hold on!'" That was my mantra. My heart and nerve and sinew were only hanging on because of sheer will. Rudyard Kipling must have known a thing or two about endurance.

I had not seen Lance since we finished biking together. Much like on the bike, I had always been waiting for him to come pulling up beside me, say a few words and then leave me in his wake. But I guess that I had somehow missed him. Which would have been easy to do since there were thousands of others out running. At least there were a few hours ago. By now though there were just a few hundred of us left out on the course. At least it felt that way. Either way, I figured Lance had probably long since enjoyed the finish line by now.

Around mile 20, there was another turn around on the road, and as soon as I made my turn I saw Lance. He was only about 50 yards behind me. I slowed down until he caught me and we jogged along together for the last six miles. I was completely shocked to discover that I had been in front of him the whole time. Turns out he was dealing with serious knee pain and had to wrestle in and out of his tri suit a few more times than me. Just the same, it was nice to have some company out there for a change. Volunteers handed glow sticks to all the runners to wear for safety. It was now very late.

We talked about the day, the swim, the bike and the run. We were so close to the end and we knew it. We could feel the excitement awaiting us just a few miles down the road. It was ours for the taking and we knew beyond a shadow of a doubt that we were about to take it. I had been looking at my watch and doing the math throughout the run. Just to make sure that I could still afford my walk breaks. Which by now were becoming longer and more frequent. Those aid stations were now about 13 minutes apart.

Finally, we reached mile 24 and the volunteers told us that this was the very last aid station. We decided we did not need any more walk breaks. We figured that if we picked up the pace a little bit, we might be able to finish in less than 16 hours. We agreed that a finish time that started with a 15 as opposed to a 16 would have a much better ring to it.

On the dark, quiet, lonely streets outside of Louisville,

we had not seen or heard a cheering spectator in the last hour or two. Suddenly, there were two guys in the middle of the road out in front of us just screaming to us at the top of their lungs, "You've only got two miles to go! Just two miles and you're done!" Their yell had an almost begging sound to it. They were pleading with us. Their enthusiasm was contagious and quickened our pace.

We were now in the heart of downtown and began making left turns, then right turns. We could hear the distant sound of horns and cheers. We ran faster. First he would pick up the pace and I would have to catch up. Then I would return the favor. Then we made that final turn and we could see the finish line out in front only a few city blocks away. We could hear the madness as we ran towards the lights.

{ TIP: DITCH THE GLOW STICK PRIOR TO THE FINISH LINE. YOU LOSE COOL POINTS FOR HAVING THEM IN YOUR FINISH LINE PHOTO. }

I soaked it all in with all of my might. I breathed deeply and looked around at every face and poster. I had wanted this for so long. This was the reason I took my bike on vacation and did training bricks while others slept in. This was the reason I swam laps in the dark before work. This was the moment I had worked so hard to make a reality. Then my ears focused in on the words of the announcer blasting out over the

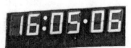

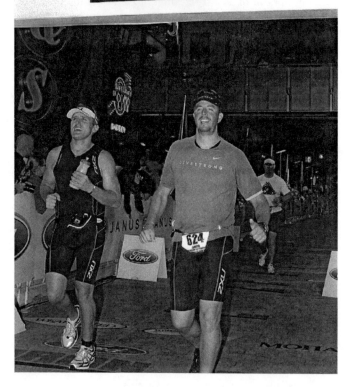

{ *There's the day you get married, the day your kids are born, and the day you finish an Ironman. Few things in life could top this moment. (We crossed that finish line with an official time of 15:58.)* }

speakers, I heard "Okinawa, Japan...US Air Force...#624 David Mills." I relished in the moment and high-fived all the out-stretched arms from the spectators that lined the road. Then Lance and I crossed the finish line together. The official time was 15:58. It has a nice ring to it, don't you think?

Someone put a finisher's medal around my neck. Another person put a blanket over my shoulders and a bottle of water in my hand. Maybe it was the endorphins or the adrenaline, I don't know, but I felt fantastic as I stood and talked and took pictures with my friends and family. It was how I imagine it feels to stand at the top of Mt. Everest.

Just three years earlier I had stood and watched as a spectator. Speechless and dumbfounded I wondered if I had it in me to do something like that. Now I was the one crossing the finish line. I like to think that maybe someone in that crowd saw me and thought, "If that guy can do it, then I surely I could too."

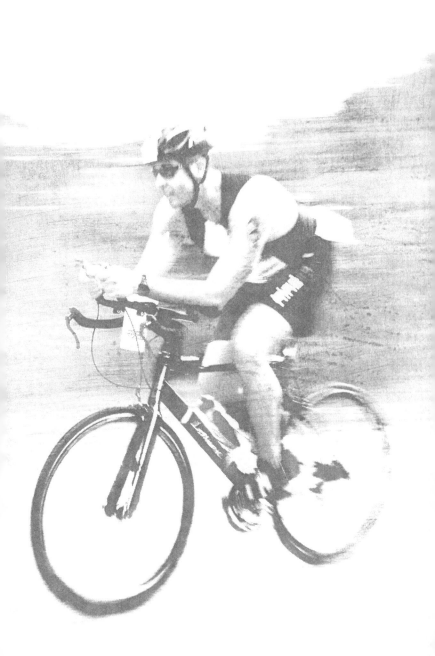

CHAPTER 19

THE AFTERMATH

"Excellence is not an act but rather a habit. We are what we repeatedly do." — Aristotle

The breakfast that I ate the next morning was the best meal of my life. We all went out to Cracker Barrel, where I ordered the country fried steak and eggs, complete with biscuits, grits and hash browns. I felt surprisingly well. I was a little sore, but nothing too extreme. Nothing that a little ibuprofen and a lot of coffee couldn't fix.

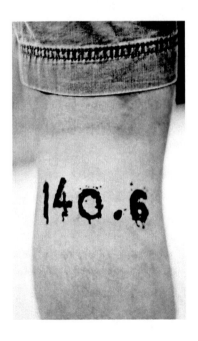

I believe that everyone has a ghost buried in their past. Something that they started that they always wish they would have finished. Or maybe something that they never even started but always wished they had. We are all haunted by some experience in our

{ *I picked a font that looked the way I felt when I finished* } past that hangs over and whispers, "You're a quitter. Remember me? You never finished me, did you?" We cannot go back in time and fix the things that we gave up on or coward away from. What's done is done. But what we can do is determine that we will never fall victim to those faults again. That we have learned from the past and that we have changed.

I can personally verify that with the completion of an Ironman comes the ultimate burial of those old ghosts. I had my list hanging over me of things I had started and never finished. That list evaporated into irrelevance the moment I crossed that finish line and heard the announcer say those magic words — "You ARE an Ironman!" I laid any haunting doubts or suspicions about what I was or was not capable of to rest. I had bit off the biggest mouthful imaginable, chewed it up, swallowed it and showed my empty mouth to the world.

If you're looking for a way to bury your own personal ghosts then believe me, the Ironman will lay them to rest. Permanently. It will cleanse your spirit. It will uncloud your mind. It will do nothing short of making you a better human. And it cannot be oversold.

It's been a year since the completion of my Ironman. My bike has gathered a bit of dust and my tri suit would be a littler bit tighter if I were to put it back on. But my mind and spirit have been forever changed. The knowledge that I can do anything I put my mind to is an incredible edge. I can do ANYTHING that I put my mind to! What a concept to believe about yourself. Sure we all hear our mothers say it to us as kids, but how many adults literally believe that about themselves. I can think of about 44,000 adults that started believing it about themselves in 2009. I'm one of them.

There are few events in life worthy of permanently inking onto your skin. The Ironman is one of them. There are tattoos for military units, motorcycle gangs, rock stars and Ironman Triathletes. These are the formidable ranks you join when you finish an Ironman.

The man who inked on my tattoo worked at Monster Ink in Okinawa, Japan. He looked like a Hell's Angel biker and was covered from head to toe in tattoos. As he worked, burning my hard-earned tattoo onto my left calf, he finally asked, "So what does this 140.6 mean?"

I explained that was the total distance of an Ironman Triathlon — 2.4-mile swim, 112-mile bike, 26.2-mile run. That I had just returned from finishing one in the States.

"You are the craziest dude that I've ever seen," he said. He called his buddy over and told me to tell him what I had just done. They couldn't believe it.

I walked out of their tattoo parlor wearing a proud smile. I had just earned the respect of a group of ink slingers. "I was on the moon!"

I'm always amazed at the range of questions people ask me about my Ironman experience. Surprisingly, two of the more common questions are, "How did I go to the bathroom?"

And, "Did I eat anything?" I always answer honestly and I never sugar coat it. "Yes, I peed on the bike while I coasted downhill, but no, I went into a port-a-potty for No. 2. And yes, I ate power bars, goo packs, bananas, peanut butter bagels and fruit throughout the entire race — even a cherry pie!" Of all the difficulties that I overcame in swimming, biking and running for 140.6 miles and all that people want to know about is eating and using the bathroom! I bet astronauts get that too. They travel into space. They stand on the moon. They experience and accomplish things that most people will only dream about. Then they get asked questions about Tang.

Sometimes I think about that Saturday Night Live sketch and I laugh to myself. I find myself in the supermarket thinking, "I've finished an Ironman!" That feeling that you've done something so incredible that it is not of this world is something that I think every Ironman can relate to. It will be the greatest accomplishment of your life. It will change the way you look at yourself in the mirror. You'll feel like you've been to the moon.

(Lance called again the other day. He's talking about climbing Mt. Everest.)

{ ACKNOWLEDGEMENTS }

No part of my training, traveling, competing or writing would have been possible without my amazing wife Kerry. Even though I initially registered for the Ironman against her better judgment, she quickly threw her full support behind me. Thanks Kerry, for being such an encouragement through my training, and such a good listener as I began to write it all down.

To Luke and Braeden for your sheer excitement when you found out that I was writing a book, and for always asking me how my workout went.

I will also be forever amazed by my sisters Amy, Kathryn and Donna, my parents and life-long friend Drew Richards for traveling all the way to Louisville to cheer me on. You stood for 16 hours and followed me throughout the entire day. Your encouragement and praise fueled me! Without you it would have been a very lonely and monotonous day. You made it unforgettable. A special thanks to the entire Payne family — you made me feel like one of your own, whether in Jersey, Corolla or Louisville. Thanks! And to Lance Payne, for convincing me to register for the Ironman, I would not have bitten off such an enormous undertaking without your egging me on. We did it, man!

Thanks also to the incredible men and women of the 82d Reconnaissance Squadron who followed my race online from the other side of the world. Thanks for your support, motivation and karaoke!

And to Jeffrey Jeffords, pastor of Longleaf Church in Warner Robins, Georgia for your great ideas and encouragement over countless cups of coffee at Bare Bulb Coffee. And a special thanks to Sean Cooper of Cooper Productions for making the video trailers.

Lastly, I have to thank the Japanese gentleman who returned to see if I was okay after he hit me with his car. Thanks for giving me a ride back to the Air Force base and for buying me new wheels for my bike. Arigato!

{ ABOUT THE AUTHOR }

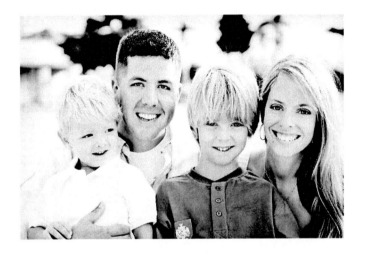

David Mills and his wife Kerry live in Georgia with their two sons Luke and Braeden. When he's not taking his kids to ball practice or navigating jets for the Air Force, he avidly pursues his passions of backpacking, reading and drinking coffee. As of the publishing of this book, David is deployed to the Middle East where he is training for his second Ironman. (Yes, he brought his bike.)

You can contact David at TheAverageIronman@gmail.com, or visit his website www.TheDistanceBook.com. He loves to hear from his readers, because after all, he is an Average Joe.

CPSIA information can be obtained at www.ICGtesting.com
Printed in the USA
LVOW090525240312

274605LV00001B/5/P

9 781935 986102